INFLAMMATION RESEARCH PERSPECTIVES

INFLAMMATION RESEARCH PERSPECTIVES

GIOCOMO T. ROMANO
EDITOR

Nova Biomedical Books
New York

For permission to use material from this book please contact us:
Telephone 631-231-7269; Fax 631-231-8175
Web Site: http://www.novapublishers.com

LIBRARY OF CONGRESS CATALOGING-IN-PUBLICATION DATA

Inflammation research perspectives / Giocomo T. Romano (editor).
p. ; cm.
Includes bibliographical references and index.
ISBN-13: 978-1-60021-845-3 (hardcover)
ISBN-10: 1-60021-845-8 (hardcover)
1. Inflammation. I. Romano, Giocomo T.
[DNLM: 1. Inflammation. QZ 150 I4365 2007]
RB131.I547 2007
616'.0473--dc22

2007034875

Published by Nova Science Publishers, Inc. ✦ New York

CONTENTS

PREFACE

Inflammation is the complex biological response of vascular tissues to harmful stimuli, such as pathogens, damaged cells, or irritants. It is a protective attempt by the organism to remove the injurious stimuli as well as initiate the healing process for the tissue. Inflammation is not a synonym for infection. Even in cases where inflammation is caused by infection it is incorrect to use the terms as synonyms: infection is caused by an exogenous pathogen, while inflammation is the response of the organism to the pathogen.

In the absence of inflammation, wounds and infections would never heal and progressive destruction of the tissue would compromise the survival of the organism. However, inflammation which runs unchecked can also lead to a host of diseases, such as hay fever, atherosclerosis, and rheumatoid arthritis. It is for this reason that inflammation is normally tightly regulated by the body.

Inflammation can be classified as either acute or chronic. Acute inflammation is the initial response of the body to harmful stimuli and is achieved by the increased movement of plasma and leukocytes from the blood into the injured tissues. A cascade of biochemical events propagates and matures the inflammatory response, involving the local vascular system, the immune system, and various cells within the injured tissue. Prolonged inflammation, known as chronic inflammation, leads to a progressive shift in the type of cells which are present at the site of inflammation and is characterised by simultaneous destruction and healing of the tissue from the inflammatory process.

Chapter I - Astrocytes perform many critical functions in the central nervous system. While their role in metabolism and maintenance of the extracellular fluid ionic composition was recognized long ago, additional roles in regulation of neurotransmitters and synaptic function have been recognized more recently. Astrocyte activation with injury and inflammation was initially recognized on morphological grounds. Recent work has begun to clarify the signaling molecules- including chemokines, cytokines, and oxidative species that astrocytes release and to which they can respond. Furthermore, as inflammation is an important feature of many neurodegenerative diseases, the ability of astrocytes to participate in inflammation is an area that is receiving increasing attention. The authors review astrocyte function relevant to inflammation, and conclude with a consideration of the role of astrocytes in inflammation following ischemic brain injury and in multiple sclerosis.

Chapter II - The role of endothelial dysfunction and endovascular inflammation in the etiology of many disease states is in the process of being unravelled.The metabolic syndrome, type 2 diabetes, obesity, and related conditions have a common underlying pathophysiology of insulin resistance, vasculo-endothelial abnormalities, and a heightened proinflammatory state. A wealth of recent evidence shows that elevated levels of various inflammatory markers are associated with the presence and severity of these pathophysiologic processes, and may, to some extent, serve as mediators in a chronic atherosclerotic disease setting. C-reactive protein is the most extensively studied of these substances, but the list includes of postulated markers includes a whole host of other molecules like interleukin-1 and the adipocytokines. Investigation into their possible role in contributing to adverse clinical outcomes has generated intense excitement, making them targets of future therapeutic modalities. Improved understanding of these markers promises to enhance the authors efforts at prevention and treatment of these states of insulin resisitance.

Chapter III - A network of microglial cells extends throughout the central nervous system (CNS) forming a ubiquitous system of endogenous immunocompetent cells (Graeber & Streit, 1990). This pervasive system ensures that every part of the CNS is under continuous surveillance and that any disturbance in homeostasis, regardless of its location, receives immediate attention for it is the role of microglia to provide a first line of defense in response to any kind of acute perturbation or injury. Inflammation is the tissue response to injury, and microglia represent the principal parenchymal cell type involved in the neuroinflammation that occurs inevitably as a result of acute CNS tissue injury. Often an injury, such as trauma or ischemia, directly causes irreversible tissue necrosis that can produce large amounts of tissue debris. Removal of tissue debris is *the* primary and undisputable function of microglial cells, which provide a quintessential source of endogenous CNS macrophages. This appreciation of microglia as brain macrophages has a long history dating as far back as the beginning of the 20th century (Barron, 1995), and it is probably fair to say that the macrophage identity is one of the few facts that is beyond debate when it comes to microglial cell functions. Other aspects of microglial biology have been more controversial, for example, the question of ontogeny, i.e. whether the cells derive from mesoderm or neuroectoderm, was debated for decades but appears to have been resolved in favor of mesoderm (Streit, 2001).

Chapter IV - Both traumatic brain injury (TBI) and spinal cord injury (SCI) are devastating conditions and leading causes of death and severe disability among young individuals. During the acute phase of injury, the primary mechanical impact to the brain or spinal cord induces an immediate tissue disruption causing focal hemorrhage, edema, release of excitatory amino acids and oxygen radicals. As a consequence of these initial events, a phase of secondary damage is initiated, during which neurochemical and metabolic alterations take place at the cellular level, ultimately leading to diffuse cell death and, often, tissue cavitation (in the spinal cord particularly, Hausmann, 2003). The inflammatory response is activated and the initial lesion expands as the injury progresses into a chronic phase. This inflammatory response is sustained by the concerted action of both peripheral cells (neutrophils, macrophages and lymphocytes) infiltrating the central nervous system (CNS) through a compromised blood brain barrier (BBB), and resident cells, particularly astrocytes and microglia. In these cell populations, which can be considered the resident inflammatory cells of the CNS, proinflammatory signal transduction cascades, such as the NF-κB pathway, are promptly activated following injury. This leads to the synthesis and release of cytokines, chemokines, extracellular matrix molecules, prostanoids, nitric oxide (NO), etc., which sustain and amplify the inflammatory reaction resulting in additional tissue loss.

The aim of this review is to discuss the contribution of glial cells to the inflammatory response of the CNS to neurotrauma, based on the vast body of data accumulated from in vivo models of TBI as well as SCI.

Chapter V - This chapter summerizes the complex interactions of immune cells and mediators in developing ischemic brain lesions and reviews current concepts on their role in neurotoxicity and –protection.

Inflammation has so far mainly been studied in the context of autoimmunity and infections of the nervous system. Only recently it has been recognized that inflammatory responses which involve hematogenous leukocytes, local microglia and immune mediators exert important functions in the pathophysiology of cerebral ischemia, a primarily non-immune lesion paradigm. Cerebral ischemia leads to immediate activation of microglia and to a temporarily graded infiltration of granulocytes, T-cells, and finally macrophages. Early microglial activation is accompanied by the upregulation of cytokines in ischemic brain lesions, and cellular adhesion molecules on corresponding endothelial cells within hours. Attenuation of microglial responses and blocking of immune mediators ameliorate ischemic brain injury in some settings suggesting a detrimental role in infarct development. Tumor necrosis factor (TNF)-alpha, members of the interleukin (IL)-1 family, and nitric oxide have been identified as main players in delayed neuronal cell death. In contrast to granulocytes and lymphocytes, macrophage entry into ischemic lesions appears to be delayed as revealed in vivo by iron contrast-enhanced magnetic resonance imaging (MRI). Thus, macrophages play a major role in tissue remodelling rather than injury.

Surprisingly, inflammation also confers neuroprotection in the brain. After hypoxic or chemical preconditioning rendering neurons less susceptible to subsequent hypoxemia, neuroprotective effects are mediated by cytokines and hematopoietic growth factors. Similarly manipulating the immune system by oral or nasal toleralization against myelin and cell adhesion proteins protects against ischemic brain injury. These beneficial effects are transferable to naive animals by T-cells.

Chapter VI - The hallmarks of inflammation were described some 2000 years ago by Cornelius Celsus as "rubor et tumor cum calore et dolore" meaning "redness and swelling with heat and pain". In the 19th century this definition was extended by "functio laesa" (loss of function). This chapter provides the updated state of knowledge concerning major cellular and molecular mechanisms of this process, with a special emphasis on early events of acute inflammation: changes in a vascular permeability, formation of chemotactic gradient, and a local accumulation of inflammatory cells and molecules. The role of mast cells, macrophages and neutrophils is highlighted, and special attention is given to the soluble mediators of inflammation, such as histamine, kinins, acute phase proteins, lipid mediators, chemokines, metalloproteinases and proinflammatory cytokines, including anti-nociceptive endogenous opioids. Cytokines produced during inflammation act not only locally but also affect the central nervous system and induce changes called "sickness behaviour": depress animal mobility, exploration of physical and social environment, reduce food and water intake, and impair learning and memory.

In this chapter, participation of inflammation in the homeostatic system of the body is illustrated by the results obtained by our group during studies on peritoneal inflammation induced in representatives of mammals, amphibians, and fish. Experimental peritonitis is a very convenient model for the precise quantitative analysis of inflammatory cells and soluble factors that may be easily washed out from the inflamed peritoneal cavity of vertebrate animals. The course of inflammation depends on the kind and dose of stimulus applied, and on the investigated animals. Moreover, it may differ between animals matched according to strain, gender, and age due to some common laboratory practices such as handling, injections, or social stress such as isolation or grouping. In ectothermic vertebrates, the course of inflammation is modified by ambient temperature and season, which indicates its dependence on the annual endogenous rhythms of the body. Supplementation of inflammation-inducing agent with morphine abolishes pain, and reduces influx of leukocytes into peritoneal cavity as well as levels of plasma chemotactic factors in fish (salmon and goldfish) and several (but not all) strains of mice but in none of the investigated amphibian species. Time-dependent changes of cells and molecules in the focus of inflammation are accompanied by the pronounced changes of animal behaviour (pain symptoms) and levels of mediators (corticosteroids, endogenous opioids).

In: Inflammation Research Perspectives
Editor: Giacomo T. Romano, pp. 1-15
ISBN: 978-1-60021-845-3

Chapter I

THE CENTRAL NERVOUS SYSTEM AND INFLAMMATION: ASTROCYTES

Valerie Chock and Rona Giffard
Departments of Anesthesia and Neonatology, Stanford University School of Medicine, Stanford, CA 94305, USA.

ABSTRACT

Astrocytes perform many critical functions in the central nervous system. While their role in metabolism and maintenance of the extracellular fluid ionic composition was recognized long ago, additional roles in regulation of neurotransmitters and synaptic function have been recognized more recently. Astrocyte activation with injury and inflammation was initially recognized on morphological grounds. Recent work has begun to clarify the signaling molecules- including chemokines, cytokines, and oxidative species that astrocytes release and to which they can respond. Furthermore, as inflammation is an important feature of many neurodegenerative diseases, the ability of astrocytes to participate in inflammation is an area that is receiving increasing attention. We review astrocyte function relevant to inflammation, and conclude with a consideration of the role of astrocytes in inflammation following ischemic brain injury and in multiple sclerosis.

1. INTRODUCTION

Astrocytes have many roles in the central nervous system. In addition to their role in the establishment, maintenance and function of synapses, the production of neurotrophic factors, and the antioxidant defense of the brain, astrocytes are essential to establish and maintain the blood brain barrier and function as primary inflammatory cells. As inflammatory cells, astrocytes may be neuroprotective by promoting tissue repair and containing further injury, or they may be detrimental by contributing to delayed oxidative injury and upregulation of inflammatory processes. In this chapter, we examine astrocyte function in the context of inflammation and describe the contribution of astrocytes to several inflammatory disease processes. In particular we will consider the role of astrocytes in inflammation during neurodegeneration.

2. Inflammatory Response of Astrocytes in the CNS

2.1. Morphological Activation

Astrocyte activation results in cytoplasmic hypertrophy and proliferation. A key ultrastructural change is the cytoplasmic accumulation of intermediate filaments including glial fibrillary acidic protein (GFAP). Reactive astrocytes, such as those seen following both global and focal ischemia, exhibit more intense GFAP-staining, thickened cellular processes and evidence of hypertophy (Figure 1, 2A). Activation also includes reexpression of nestin, characteristic of intermediate filaments in immature astrocytes but generally undetectable in adult brain (Figure 2B). In addition, astrocytes display increased nuclear size and an increased number of mitochondria, ribosomes, and Golgi complexes [12]; for review see [56]. They are poised for increased production of numerous molecules involved in inflammation including cytokines, chemokines, nitric oxide synthase, metalloproteinases, and intracellular adhesion molecules.

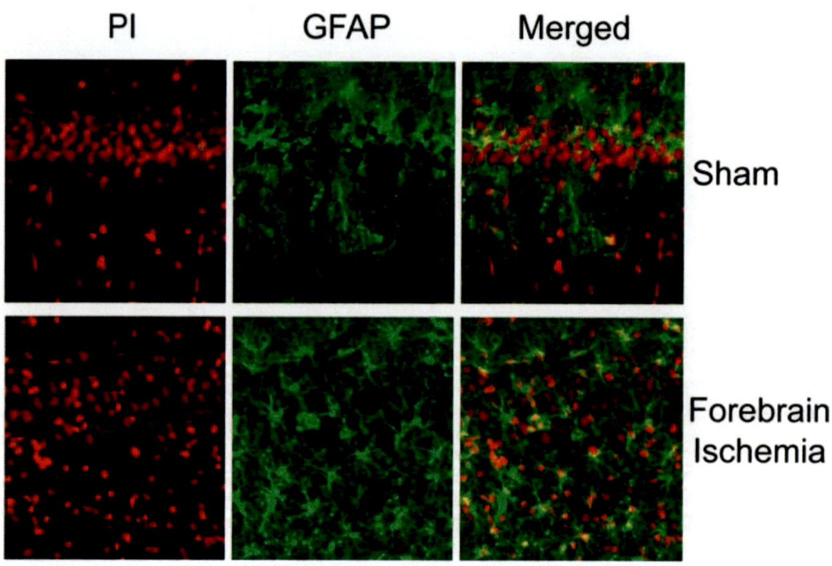

Figure 1. GFAP staining 72 hours following transient global ischemia reveals astrocyte activation in the hippocampus. Rats were subjected to bilateral carotid artery occlusion and hypotension for 10 minutes, followed by reperfusion (forebrain ischemia) or sham operation without ischemia. The animals was sacrificed 72 hours later and frozen sections were stained with anti-GFAP antibody and visualized with fluorescent secondary antibody (green). Red is propidium iodide to show nuclei. The dense horizontal band of nuclei visible in the upper left panel shows the level of the CA1 neuronal cell bodies. By 72

hours many of these neurons are lost, lower left panel, while the level of GFAP expression and the size of astrocytes is clearly increased.

2.2. Production of Cytokines

The presence of cytokines in the CNS has been attributed not only to invading leukocytes and macrophages, but also to resident glial cells. Astrocytes have been shown to produce a variety of cytokines under pathologic conditions (see Table 1). These include IL-1α, IL-1β, IL-6, IL-10, IFN-α, IFN-β, IFN-γ, TNF-α, TGF-β, GM-CSF, M-CSF, and G-CSF as observed

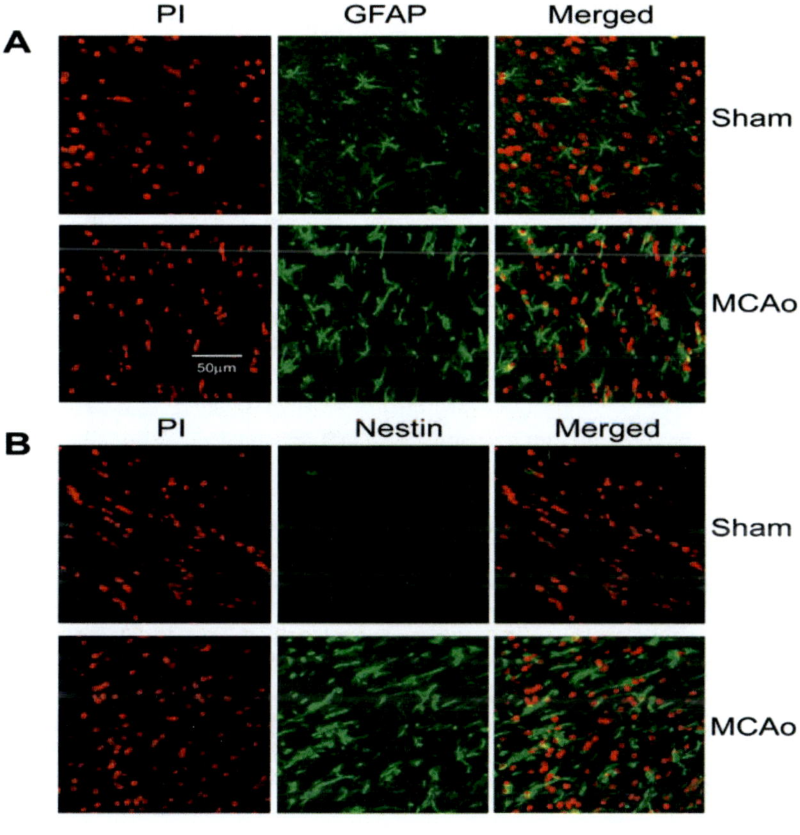

Figure 2. Changes in GFAP and nestin staining 72 hours following transient focal ischemia. Rats were subjected to suture occlusion of the middle cerebral artery for 2 hours followed by reperfusion (MCAO), and sacrificed at 72 hours. A. Sections were stained with anti-GFAP antibody and detected with fluorescent secondary antibody (green). Sham animals were not subjected to suture occlusion. Propidium iodide was used as a counterstain to show the nuclei. Increased GFAP staining is seen with relative thickening of astrocytic processes. B. Sections were stained with anti-nestin antibody (detected as green fluorescence) and counterstained with propidium iodide. In the sham animal no nestin immunoreactivity is detected, while after MCAO there is marked upregulation of nestin in astrocytes.

in both *in vitro* and *in vivo* investigations (for reviews see [18,23]. Each cytokine in turn can cause a myriad of effects. For example, IL-1 is a potent mitogen for astrocytes and induces release of neuronal growth factor from astrocytes. IL-6 also promotes astrogliosis, modulates neurotransmitter biosynthesis, and protects neurons against ischemic injury (for review see [30].

Production of specific cytokines may be induced or inhibited by other cytokines previously released by activated microglia or other astrocytes in a paracrine feedback loop. Bacterial products alone such as lipopolysaccharide (LPS) are sufficient to stimulate astrocyte production of cytokines including IL-1β and TNFα [15,28,38] and IL-6 [5,28] in cultured astrocytes. Astrocytes recognize bacterial products via their expression of toll-like receptors (TLRs), which are microbial pattern-recognition receptors. Cultured astrocytes express a number of different TLRs which increase after exposure to LPS and other bacterial ligands, resulting in activation of the transcription factor NF-κB and subsequent synthesis of pro-inflammatory cytokines like IL-6 [9].

2.3. Production of Chemokines

Similar to microglia, astrocytes also produce chemokines, a class of chemoattractant cytokines, which mediate migration of peripheral immune cells into the CNS. Astrocytes have been shown to produce RANTES, IL-8, MCP-1, and IP-10 (for reviews see [18,23]. In response to the proinflammatory cytokines TNF-α, IFN-γ, or IL-1β, astrocytes are the major producers of the chemokine MCP-1. This chemokine, which is often identified in the perivascular space, binds the CCR2 receptor on endothelial cells [70] as well as binding receptors on peripheral blood monocytes and activated T-cells to induce migration of these leukocytes across the blood-brain barrier. [76]. MCP-1 is expressed by astrocytes during flares of experimental autoimmune encephalomyelitis (EAE) [26] whereas MCP-1 deficient mice are resistant to EAE [35]. MCP-1 expression has also been localized to astrocytes during traumatic brain injury [24]. MCP-1 acting via the CCR2 receptor has been shown to increase blood brain barrier leakiness and increase edema, an effect missing in CCR2 knockout mice [70].

2.4. Astrocytes as Antigen Presenting Cells (APCs)

The ability of astrocytes to function as APCs is controversial. Typical antigen presenting cells like B-cells and macrophages normally express major histocompatibility complex (MHC) class II molecules, which allow presentation of processed antigens to $CD4^+$ T-helper cells with subsequent T-cell activation and induction of an immune response. However, expression of MHC class II can be induced on astrocytes and is regulated by various cytokines and neuropeptides [18]. For example, interferon-γ is the most potent inducer of class II MHC expression on astrocytes [78], while TNF-α enhances IFN-γ-induced expression of class II MHC, but alone has no effect [55]. Inhibitors of class II MHC expression on astrocytes include TGF-β, IFN-β, IL-1, IL-4, norepinephrine, glutamate, nitric oxide, and vasoactive intestinal peptide [18].

Class II MHC expressing astrocytes have been shown to process and present antigens and activate both naïve and memory T cells [52,68]. In contrast, other investigators have shown that class II MHC expressing astrocytes are not capable of stimulating T-cell proliferation and instead induce apoptosis or down-regulation of T cells [47,75]. Such a response may be beneficial for astrocyte suppression of CNS autoimmunity like in multiple sclerosis. The absence of costimulatory molecule expression on astrocytes (B7 or CD40) may be responsible for the variability in astrocyte response [27,62]. Other studies further suggest that astrocyte activation of T-cells can only occur after priming by microglia [67,77]. Therefore, the ability of astrocytes to function as antigen presenting cells with ensuing T-cell proliferation or suppression may depend on the setting and awaits further clarification.

2.5. Production of iNOS/ Nitric Oxide

Exposure to bacterial endotoxin and various cytokines including IFN-γ results in inducible nitric oxide synthase (iNOS) production and subsequent nitric oxide (NO) release from both astrocytes and microglia [10]. Cultured astrocytes, moreover, were found to increase iNOS 96-fold after exposure to LPS and IFN-γ [7]. Generated nitric oxide can diffuse to and injure surrounding cells. Nitric oxide and its toxic metabolite, peroxynitrite, can inhibit components of the mitochondrial respiratory chain, leading to cellular energy deficiency and eventual cell death. Neuronal ATP loss [34] and mitochondrial damage [3] have been reported in cocultures of neurons and iNOS-producing astrocytes. Therefore, decreasing nitric oxide production by astrocytes is a potential neuroprotective strategy. Complicating the picture is the role of astrocytes in protecting neurons from oxidative stress, including potentially that induced by NO. Astrocytes have higher intracellular levels of the antioxidant glutathione, they are less vulnerable to oxidative injury than neurons, and have also been shown to protect neurons from NO [13]. In response to prolonged exposure to NO astrocytes can upregulate glutamate-cysteine ligase, the rate-limiting enzyme in GSH synthesis, while neurons appear unable to do this [22].

2.6. Maintenance of the Blood Brain Barrier

The blood brain barrier (BBB) consists of a continuous capillary endothelium with tight junctions between cells. Astrocytes and microglia cover approximately 85% of the endothelial surface, with astrocyte foot processes in close apposition to the microvascular endothelium (for reviews see [4,33]. At the BBB interface astrocytes and microglia interact with each other and with peripheral inflammatory cells via cytokines, influencing entry of inflammatory cells into the brain. Interactions between astrocytes and endothelial cells are essential to the integrity of the BBB and modulate endothelial cell function. For example, astrocytes increase electrical resistance across cultured endothelial cells and enhance their intercellular connections [40]. Ablation of astrocytes led to failure of BBB repair and vasogenic edema [11]. Selective ablation of reactive astrocytes in the setting of spinal cord injury in a transgenic mouse model also resulted in failure of BBB repair, augmented leukocyte infiltration, neuronal and oligodendrocyte death, and pronounced motor deficits [20]. Astrocytes are important in maintaining BBB integrity in disease states. Disruption of this barrier leads to edema and increased access of peripheral immune cells and humoral factors to the central nervous system. Astrocytes also can express metalloproteinases (MMPs) and intercellular adhesion molecules (ICAMs) upon activation. Specifically, MMP-9 is produced by activated astrocytes and acts as an extracellular matrix collagenase, contributing to BBB breakdown [29]. ICAM-1 is expressed by activated astrocytes in response to TNF-α, IFN-γ, and TLR ligands *in vitro* and *in vivo* and can contribute to the recruitment and further invasion of circulating immune cells [23,42] into the CNS. As noted above, MCP-1 is also produced by astrocytes and plays a role in both blood brain barrier permeability and recruitment of peripheral monocytes [70].

3. Regulators of Astrocyte Inflammatory Function

IL-1β has been shown to play a central role in regulating the reactive response of astrocytes via Rho signaling pathways [37]. The transcription factor NF-κB is persistently activated in response to cerebral ischemia, proinflammatory stimuli, and reactive oxygen species. In astrocytes and microglia, activated NF-κB can induce expression of other inflammatory genes such as iNOS, matrix metalloproteinase-9, COX-2, leukocyte adhesion molecules, and proinflammatory cytokines, eventually leading to breakdown of the blood-brain barrier and the generation of neurotoxic reactive oxygen species [49]. Much still remains to be learned about the regulation of gene expression during inflammatory activation of astrocytes.

3.1. Response to Cytokines/ Chemokines

Not only do astrocytes produce cytokines and chemokines, their production of these factors is in itself regulated by the presence of other cytokines. *In vivo* injection of TNF-α into mouse brain resulted in upregulation of RANTES and MIP-1α [25]. TNF-α production by astrocytes is induced by IFN-γ, IL-1, and TNF-α, but inhibited by IL-6, IL-10, and TGF-β. Astrocytic release of IL-6 is induced by TNF-α, IFN-γ, TGF-β, and IL-1, for review see [18]. There is thus a complex interplay of autocrine and paracrine effects of cytokines between astrocytes and microglia that determine the final responses of these cells as well as their activity as sources of these regulatory molecules. For a partial list of some inducers and inhibitors of astrocyte cytokine expression see Table 1.

Table 1. Cytokines produced by astrocytes

Molecule	Inducers	Inhibitors
GM-CSF	TNF-α, IL-1	TGF-β
IL-6	TNF-α, IFN-γ, TGF-β, IL-1	
TNF-α	IFN-γ, IL-1, TNF-α	TGF-β, IL-6, IL-10
TGF-β	IL-1, TGF-β	
MCP-1	TNF-α, IFN-γ, IL-1, TGF-β, Fas ligation, HIV-1 Tat	
RANTES	TNF-α, IL-1	
IP-10	TNF-α, IFN-γ, HIV-1 Tat, Fas ligation	

GM-CSF, granulocyte/macrophage colony-stimulating factor; IL-1, -6, -10, interleukin-1, -6, -10; TNF-α, tumor necrosis factor-α; TGF, transforming growth factor; IFN-γ, interferon-γ; HIV-1, human immunodeficiency virus type 1.

Table from Dong and Benveniste, 2001, Glia 36:180, used with permission.

3.2. Complement

Complement also activates astrocytes. Complement receptors for C3a and C5a are expressed on astrocytes and when activated lead to increased intracellular calcium via the phospholipase C pathway as well as activation of the MAPK pathway [65]. Following exposure to C3a and C5a anaphylatoxins, human astrocytes *in vitro* have shown increased IL-6 mRNA expression which may be neuroprotective [57,64], and may facilitate increased IL-8 expression [36]. Recent work supports a role for a novel C5a receptor isoform on astrocytes with anti-inflammatory properties [21]. Complement may also play a role in mediating excitotoxic neuronal death through astrocytes [72]. Both C1q and C3 can be made by astrocytes [69], so as with cytokines, astrocytes have a dynamic role both producing and responding to complement, which also interacts with cytokine responses.

3.3. Interaction with Microglia

Microglia actively monitor the brain even while in their resting state [53]. However, recent work suggests that purinergic signaling by astrocytes may be involved in the earliest responses of microglia to injury [16]. ATP, at least in part released by astrocytes, was shown to alter microglial dynamics, including in the setting of acute injury [16]. Thus astrocytes may in some cases be the first responders which then recruit microglia. Microglia as sensors and early responders to injury, can secrete proinflammatory cytokines such as IL-1b and TNF-α that can then activate adjacent astrocytes and microglia by autocrine and paracrine pathways, thus resulting in propagation of the inflammatory response. For review see [61]. Astrocytes in turn can stimulate microglial proliferation and activation *in vitro* through the production of M-CSF [31] and laminin [45]. Microglia may have a synergistic inflammatory effect with astrocytes. In an *in vitro* model of the blood brain barrier exposed to ischemia-like conditions, co-cultures of brain endothelial cells and astrocytes exhibited markedly greater injury when microglia were plated with the other two cell types [80]. However, others have found a more protective role for interacting microglia and astrocytes. Microglia-derived GDNF protects astrocytes in culture from ischemia-like injury [43]. Also, microglia *in vitro* survived ischemia-like injury better in the presence of astrocytes [74]. See chapter 2 this volume by Streit et al. for a discussion of the beneficial effects of microglia and an in depth discussion of microglia activation.

3.4. Developmental Changes in Astrocyte Inflammatory Response

Little work has been done on glial inflammatory responses in the context of development. We have found that microglia cultured for a short time are more sensitive to ischemia-like injury *in vitro* than those cultured for longer durations, and may contribute to worsening brain injury by increased release of the inflammatory cytokines TNF-α and IL-1β [14]. Early differentiating oligodendrocytes are also more vulnerable to free radical injury and cytokine injury compared to mature oligodendrocytes [1,2]. However, similar exploration of astrocytic inflammatory changes with development still needs investigation. Age-specific changes occur with astrocyte expression of apoptotic mediators. Primary astrocytes cultured for short times undergo more apoptosis after serum deprivation and have higher levels of the pro-apoptotic protein bax and greater ERK kinase expression compared astrocytes cultured for longer durations [79]. Blood brain barrier breakdown after an excitotoxic lesion in juvenile rats resulted in greater leukocyte recruitment compared to adult rats [8], potentially reflecting changing astrocytic response in BBB maintenance with age. On the opposite end of the age spectrum, a model of traumatic brain injury in aged rats showed exacerbated glial activation and enhanced release of the inflammatory cytokines Il-1β, TNF-α, IL-6, ICAM-1, iNOS, and MMP-9 compared to young rats [41].

Clinical studies further demonstrate developmental variation in glial responses. Pathology data from the National Collaborative Perinatal Project showed that in preterm infants, periventricular leukomalacia, a debilitating white matter injury, peaked at 32-35 weeks' gestation while hypertrophic astrocytes peaked at 36-44 weeks' gestation [44]. This correlation of change in astrocyte response with reduced susceptibility is suggestive. Developmental differences in astrocytic response to insult may account for some of the variation in outcomes at different gestational ages. Similarly with regards to the aged population, chronic inflammation and production of pro-inflammatory cytokines by astrocytes and microglia may in part contribute to amyloid formation and the pathogenesis of Alzheimer's disease [32,48].

4. Specific Neurological Diseasesand Astrocyte Activation

The role of astrocytes and inflammation in stroke, Alzheimer's disease, Parkinson's disease, and trauma is reviewed in greater detail elsewhere [84]. We briefly discuss astrocyte inflammatory involvement during the pathologic processes of ischemia and multiple sclerosis here.

4.1. Ischemia

Astrocytes may serve both protective and destructive roles during cerebral ischemia. Astrocytes play a crucial role in antioxidant defenses. Astrocytes have more glutathione and are more resistant to oxidative injury [6]. Astrocytes also express the metal-binding proteins metallothionein I and II which suppress metal-catalyzed free-radical production and can scavenge reactive oxygen species [51,63]. Neurons co-cultured with astrocytes were protected from nitric oxide-induced injury by enhanced astrocytic glutathione levels [13]. Moreover, neuronal glutathione concentration was found to double after 24 hours of co-culturing with astrocytes [34]. Thus, astrocytes can upregulate neuronal antioxidant capability in addition to actively detoxifying reactive oxygen species in the brain. Furthermore, glutamate excitotoxicity after ischemia can be modulated by astrocytic clearance of glutamate. Neuronal vulnerability to glutamate was 100-fold greater in astrocyte-poor cultures in comparison to cultures with abundant astrocytes [19,60]. In addition, neuronal growth factors like BDNF, EGF, NGF, and FGF are released by reactive astrocytes and may contribute to synaptogenesis and neurogenesis after ischemia [66,71]. Astrocytes also release neuropilin and VEGF which may promote angiogenesis after cerebral ischemia [39,83], although VEGF is also associated with increased vascular permeability and could contribute to edema formation [58].

In contrast, astrocytes may have detrimental effects after ischemia. Increased NO production after ischemia may lead to decreased glutamine synthase activity by astrocytes, decreased glutamate uptake, and subsequent glutamate neurotoxicity [7,50]. Activated astrocytes after ischemia also produce numerous inflammatory cytokines with pleiotropic effects including thrombosis, demyelination, and BBB disruption [18]. As noted above, MCP-1 may be another mediator released by astrocytes which could modulate BBB function and increase edema in the setting of ischemia [70]. Rat brain astrocytes were found to have increased MMP-2 activity after ischemia, which correlated with increased BBB permeability [59]. Furthermore, investigators have shown that activation of cultured astrocytes by LPS and IFN-γ led to increased induction of iNOS and production of NO. After this glial activation, increased glutamate-mediated neuronal death occurred only when combined with hypoxic conditions, illustrating the synergistic effect of inflammation with ischemia. [46].

4.2. Multiple Sclerosis

Multiple sclerosis is a chronic inflammatory demyelinating disease of the central nervous system in which glial cells play a prominent role. In murine experimental autoimmune encephalomyelitis (EAE), an established animal model of multiple sclerosis, astrocyte hypertrophy coincided with manifestation of axonal damage [73]. Astrocytes in multiple sclerosis plaques produce IL-6 [54], lack β-2 adrenergic receptors, and potentially serve as antigen-presenting cells [82], thus facilitating T-cell invasion and activation. Repeated exposure of these astrocytes to inflammatory cytokines triggers unregulated inflammatory responses and increased noradrenalin levels, leading to focal areas of myelin and axonal damage [17,81].

5. Conclusion

The role of astrocytes as primary inflammatory cells in the brain is now well-established. Recent results suggest that they are among the first cells in the brain to react to an insult and activate other cells including microglia. Future investigations are imperative to clarify the complex interactions of astrocytes with other CNS cell types in normal brain function and in pathologic conditions. New studies will identify areas in which astrocyte function can be enhanced or suppressed for neuroprotection.

Acknowledgements

We would like to thank Andrew Morrow for help preparing the manuscript, Drs. Yibing Ouyang and Grace Sun for the photomicrographs. This work was supported in part by NIH grants NS37520, NS14543, and GM49831.

References

[1] Back, S.A., et al., Maturation-dependent vulnerability of oligodendrocytes to oxidative stress-induced death caused by glutathione depletion. *J Neurosci*, 1998. 18(16): p. 6241-53.

[2] Baerwald, K.D. and B. Popko, Developing and mature oligodendrocytes respond differently to the immune cytokine interferon-gamma. *J Neurosci Res*, 1998. 52(2): p. 230-9.

[3] Bal-Price, A. and G.C. Brown, Inflammatory neurodegeneration mediated by nitric oxide from activated glia-inhibiting neuronal respiration, causing glutamate release and excitotoxicity. *J Neurosci*, 2001. 21(17): p. 6480-91.

[4] Ballabh, P., A. Braun, and M. Nedergaard, The blood-brain barrier: an overview: structure, regulation, and clinical implications. *Neurobiol Dis*, 2004. 16(1): p. 1-13.

[5] Benveniste, E.N., et al., Induction and regulation of interleukin-6 gene expression in rat astrocytes. *J Neuroimmunol*, 1990. 30(2-3): p. 201-12.

[6] Bolanos, J.P., et al., Effect of peroxynitrite on the mitochondrial respiratory chain: differential susceptibility of neurones and astrocytes in primary culture. *J Neurochem,* 1995. 64(5): p. 1965-72.

[7] Bolanos, J.P., et al., Nitric oxide-mediated inhibition of the mitochondrial respiratory chain in cultured astrocytes. *J Neurochem*, 1994. 63(3): p. 910-6.

[8] Bolton, S.J. and V.H. Perry, Differential blood-brain barrier breakdown and leucocyte recruitment following excitotoxic lesions in juvenile and adult rats. *Exp Neurol*, 1998. 154(1): p. 231-40.

[9] Bowman, C.C., et al., Cultured astrocytes express toll-like receptors for bacterial products. *Glia*, 2003. 43(3): p. 281-91.

[10]Brown, G.C. and A. Bal-Price, Inflammatory neurodegeneration mediated by nitric oxide, glutamate, and mitochondria. *Mol Neurobiol*, 2003. 27(3): p. 325-55.

[11]Bush, T.G., et al., Leukocyte infiltration, neuronal degeneration, and neurite outgrowth after ablation of scar-forming, reactive astrocytes in adult transgenic mice. *Neuron*, 1999. 23(2): p. 297-308.

[12]Bushong, E.A., M.E. Martone, and M.H. Ellisman, Maturation of astrocyte morphology and the establishment of astrocyte domains during postnatal hippocampal development. *Int J Dev Neurosci*, 2004. 22(2): p. 73-86.

[13]Chen, Y., et al., Astrocytes protect neurons from nitric oxide toxicity by a glutathione-dependent mechanism. *J Neurochem*, 2001. 77(6): p. 1601-10.

[14]Chock, V.Y. and R.G. Giffard, Development of neonatal murine microglia in vitro: changes in response to lipopolysaccharide and ischemia-like injury. *Pediatr Res*, 2005. 57(4): p. 475-80.

[15]Chung, I.Y. and E.N. Benveniste, Tumor necrosis factor-alpha production by astrocytes. Induction by lipopolysaccharide, IFN-gamma, and IL-1 beta. *J Immunol*, 1990. 144(8): p. 2999-3007.

[16]Davalos, D., et al., ATP mediates rapid microglial response to local brain injury in vivo. *Nat Neurosci*, 2005. 8(6): p. 752-8.

[17]De Keyser, J., et al., Astrocytes in multiple sclerosis lack beta-2 adrenergic receptors. *Neurology*, 1999. 53(8): p. 1628-33.

[18]Dong, Y. and E.N. Benveniste, Immune function of astrocytes. *Glia*, 2001. 36(2): p. 180-90.

[19]Dugan, L.L., et al., Glia modulate the response of murine cortical neurons to excitotoxicity: glia exacerbate AMPA neurotoxicity. *J Neurosci*, 1995. 15(6): p. 4545-55.

[20]Faulkner, J.R., et al., Reactive astrocytes protect tissue and preserve function after spinal cord injury. *J Neurosci*, 2004. 24(9): p. 2143-55.

[21]Gavrilyuk, V., et al., Identification of complement 5a-like receptor (C5L2) from astrocytes: characterization of anti-inflammatory properties. *J Neurochem*, 2005. 92(5): p. 1140-9.

[22]Gegg, M.E., et al., Differential effect of nitric oxide on glutathione metabolism and mitochondrial function in astrocytes and neurones: implications for neuroprotection/neurodegeneration? *J Neurochem*, 2003. 86(1): p. 228-37.

[23]Ghirnikar, R.S., Y.L. Lee, and L.F. Eng, Inflammation in traumatic brain injury: role of cytokines and chemokines. *Neurochem Res*, 1998. 23(3): p. 329-40.

[24]Glabinski, A.R., et al., Chemokine monocyte chemoattractant protein-1 is expressed by astrocytes after mechanical injury to the brain. *J Immunol*, 1996. 156(11): p. 4363-8.

[25]Glabinski, A.R., et al., TNF-alpha microinjection upregulates chemokines and chemokine receptors in the central nervous system without inducing leukocyte infiltration. *J Interferon Cytokine Res*, 2003. 23(8): p. 457-66.

[26]Glabinski, A.R., et al., Synchronous synthesis of alpha- and beta-chemokines by cells of diverse lineage in the central nervous system of mice with relapses of chronic experimental autoimmune encephalomyelitis. *Am J Pathol*, 1997. 150(2): p. 617-30.

[27]Gold, R., et al., Antigen presentation by astrocytes primes rat T lymphocytes for apoptotic cell death. A model for T-cell apoptosis in vivo. *Brain*, 1996. 119 (Pt 2): p. 651-9.

[28]Gottschall, P.E., I. Tatsuno, and A. Arimura, Regulation of interleukin-6 (IL-6) secretion in primary cultured rat astrocytes: synergism of interleukin-1 (IL-1) and pituitary adenylate cyclase activating polypeptide (PACAP). *Brain Res*, 1994. 637(1-2): p. 197-203.

[29]Gottschall, P.E. and X. Yu, Cytokines regulate gelatinase A and B (matrix metalloproteinase 2 and 9) activity in cultured rat astrocytes. *J Neurochem*, 1995. 64(4): p. 1513-20.

[30]Gruol, D.L. and T.E. Nelson, Physiological and pathological roles of interleukin-6 in the central nervous system. *Mol Neurobiol*, 1997. 15(3): p. 307-39.

[31]Hao, C., L.J. Guilbert, and S. Fedoroff, Production of colony-stimulating factor-1 (CSF-1) by mouse astroglia in vitro. *J Neurosci Res*, 1990. 27(3): p. 314-23.

[32]Harris, M.E., et al., Amyloid beta peptide (25-35) inhibits Na+-dependent glutamate uptake in rat hippocampal astrocyte cultures. *J Neurochem*, 1996. 67(1): p. 277-86.

[33]Haseloff, R.F., et al., In search of the astrocytic factor(s) modulating blood-brain barrier functions in brain capillary endothelial cells in vitro. *Cell Mol Neurobiol*, 2005. 25(1): p. 25-39.

[34]Heales, S.J. and J.P. Bolanos, Impairment of brain mitochondrial function by reactive nitrogen species: the role of glutathione in dictating susceptibility. *Neurochem Int*, 2002. 40(6): p. 469-74.

[35]Huang, D.R., et al., Absence of monocyte chemoattractant protein 1 in mice leads to decreased local macrophage recruitment and antigen-specific T helper cell type 1 immune response in experimental autoimmune encephalomyelitis. *J Exp Med*, 2001. 193(6): p. 713-26.

[36]Jauneau, A.C., et al., Complement component anaphylatoxins upregulate chemokine expression by human astrocytes. *FEBS Lett*, 2003. 537(1-3): p. 17-22.

[37]John, G.R., et al., Interleukin-1beta induces a reactive astroglial phenotype via deactivation of the Rho GTPase-Rock axis. *J Neurosci*, 2004. 24(11): p. 2837-45.

[38]Kimberlin, D.W., et al., Modulation of expression of genes involved in the inflammatory response by lipopolysaccharide and temperature in cultured human astroglial cells. *Immunol Invest*, 1995. 24(5): p. 775-85.

[39]Krum, J.M. and A. Khaibullina, Inhibition of endogenous VEGF impedes revascularization and astroglial proliferation: roles for VEGF in brain repair. *Exp Neurol*, 2003. 181(2): p. 241-57.

[40]Kuchler-Bopp, S., et al., Astrocytes induce several blood-brain barrier properties in non-neural endothelial cells. *Neuroreport*, 1999. 10(6): p. 1347-53.

[41]Kyrkanides, S., et al., Enhanced glial activation and expression of specific CNS inflammation-related molecules in aged versus young rats following cortical stab injury. *J Neuroimmunol*, 2001. 119(2): p. 269-77.

[42]Kyrkanides, S., et al., TNF alpha and IL-1beta mediate intercellular adhesion molecule-1 induction via microglia-astrocyte interaction in CNS radiation injury. *J Neuroimmunol*, 1999. 95(1-2): p. 95-106.

[43]Lee, G.A., et al., Microglia-derived glial cell line-derived neurotrophic factor could protect Sprague-Dawley rat astrocyte from in vitro ischemia-induced damage. *Neurosci Lett*, 2004. 356(2): p. 111-4.

[44]Leviton, A. and F.H. Gilles, Acquired perinatal leukoencephalopathy. *Ann Neurol*, 1984. 16(1): p. 1-8.

[45]Liesi, P., et al., Laminin is induced in astrocytes of adult brain by injury. *Embo J*, 1984. 3(3): p. 683-6.

[46]Mander, P., et al., Nitric oxide from inflammatory-activated glia synergizes with hypoxia to induce neuronal death. *J Neurosci Res*, 2005. 79(1-2): p. 208-15.

[47]Matsumoto, Y., K. Ohmori, and M. Fujiwara, Immune regulation by brain cells in the central nervous system: microglia but not astrocytes present myelin basic protein to encephalitogenic T cells under in vivo-mimicking conditions. *Immunology*, 1992. 76(2): p. 209-16.

[48]Mattson, M.P., Oxidative stress, perturbed calcium homeostasis, and immune dysfunction in Alzheimer's disease. *J Neurovirol*, 2002. 8(6): p. 539-50.

[49]Mattson, M.P. and S. Camandola, NF-kappaB in neuronal plasticity and neurodegenerative disorders. *J Clin Invest*, 2001. 107(3): p. 247-54.

[50]Muscoli, C., et al., The effect of inflammatory stimuli on NMDA-related activation of glutamine synthase in human cultured astroglial cells. *Neurosci Lett*, 2005. 373(3): p. 184-8.

[51]Nakajima, K. and K. Suzuki, Immunochemical detection of metallothionein in brain. *Neurochem Int*, 1995. 27(1): p. 73-87.

[52]Nikcevich, K.M., et al., IFN-gamma-activated primary murine astrocytes express B7 costimulatory molecules and prime naive antigen-specific T cells. *J Immunol*, 1997. 158(2): p. 614-21.

[53]Nimmerjahn, A., F. Kirchhoff, and F. Helmchen, Resting microglial cells are highly dynamic surveillants of brain parenchyma in vivo. *Science*, 2005. 308(5726): p. 1314-8.

[54]Okuda, Y., et al., The development of autoimmune encephalomyelitis provoked by myelin oligodendrocyte glycoprotein is associated with an upregulation of both proinflammatory and immunoregulatory cytokines in the central nervous system. *J Interferon Cytokine Res*, 1998. 18(6): p. 415-21.

[55]Panek, R.B., et al., Characterization of astrocyte nuclear proteins involved in IFN-gamma- and TNF-alpha-mediated class II MHC gene expression. *J Immunol*, 1994. 153(10): p. 4555-64.

[56]Panickar, K.S. and M.D. Norenberg, Astrocytes in cerebral ischemic injury: morphological and general considerations. *Glia*, 2005. 50(4): p. 287-98.

[57]Penkowa, M., et al., Astrocyte-targeted expression of interleukin-6 protects the central nervous system during neuroglial degeneration induced by 6-aminonicotinamide. *J Neurosci Res*, 2003. 73(4): p. 481-96.

[58]Proescholdt, M.A., et al., Vascular endothelial growth factor (VEGF) modulates vascular permeability and inflammation in rat brain. J Neuropathol *Exp Neurol*, 1999. 58(6): p. 613-27.

[59]Rosenberg, G.A., et al., Immunohistochemistry of matrix metalloproteinases in reperfusion injury to rat brain: activation of MMP-9 linked to stromelysin-1 and microglia in cell cultures. *Brain Res*, 2001. 893(1-2): p. 104-12.

[60]Rosenberg, P.A. and E. Aizenman, Hundred-fold increase in neuronal vulnerability to glutamate toxicity in astrocyte-poor cultures of rat cerebral cortex. *Neurosci Lett*, 1989. 103(2): p. 162-8.

[61]Rothwell, N.J. and S.J. Hopkins, Cytokines and the nervous system II: Actions and mechanisms of action. *Trends Neurosci*, 1995. 18(3): p. 130-6.

[62]Saoudi, A., et al., Prevention of experimental allergic encephalomyelitis in rats by targeting autoantigen to B cells: evidence that the protective mechanism depends on changes in the cytokine response and migratory properties of the autoantigen-specific T cells. *J Exp Med*, 1995. 182(2): p. 335-44.

[63]Sato, M. and I. Bremner, Oxygen free radicals and metallothionein. *Free Radic Biol Med*, 1993. 14(3): p. 325-37.

[64]Sayah, S., et al., Expression of cytokines by human astrocytomas following stimulation by C3a and C5a anaphylatoxins: specific increase in interleukin-6 mRNA expression. *J Neurochem*, 1999. 72(6): p. 2426-36.

[65]Sayah, S., et al., Two different transduction pathways are activated by C3a and C5a anaphylatoxins on astrocytes. *Brain Res Mol Brain Res*, 2003. 112(1-2): p. 53-60.

[66]Schwartz, J.P. and N. Nishiyama, Neurotrophic factor gene expression in astrocytes during development and following injury. *Brain Res Bull*, 1994. 35(5-6): p. 403-7.

[67]Sedgwick, J.D., et al., Major histocompatibility complex-expressing nonhematopoietic astroglial cells prime only CD8+ T lymphocytes: astroglial cells as perpetuators but not initiators of CD4+ T cell responses in the central nervous system. *J Exp Med*, 1991. 173(5): p. 1235-46.

[68]Soos, J.M., et al., Astrocytes express elements of the class II endocytic pathway and process central nervous system autoantigen for presentation to encephalitogenic T cells. *J Immunol*, 1998. 161(11): p. 5959-66.

[69]Speth, C., et al., Complement synthesis and activation in the brain of SIV-infected monkeys. *J Neuroimmunol*, 2004. 151(1-2): p. 45-54.

[70]Stamatovic, S.M., et al., Monocyte chemoattractant protein-1 regulation of blood-brain barrier permeability. *J Cereb Blood Flow Metab*, 2005. 25(5): p. 593-606.

[71]Strauss, S., et al., Increased levels of nerve growth factor (NGF) protein and mRNA and reactive gliosis following kainic acid injection into the rat striatum. *Neurosci Lett*, 1994. 168(1-2): p. 193-6.

[72]van Beek, J., et al., Complement anaphylatoxin C3a is selectively protective against NMDA-induced neuronal cell death. *Neuroreport*, 2001. 12(2): p. 289-93.

[73]Wang, D., et al., Astrocyte-associated axonal damage in pre-onset stages of experimental autoimmune encephalomyelitis. *Glia*, 2005. 51(3): p. 235-40.

[74]Wang, J.Y., et al., Production of macrophage inflammatory protein-2 following hypoxia/reoxygenation in glial cells. *Glia*, 2000. 32(2): p. 155-64.

[75]Weber, F., et al., Human astrocytes are only partially competent antigen presenting cells. Possible implications for lesion development in multiple sclerosis. *Brain*, 1994. 117 (Pt 1): p. 59-69.

[76]Weiss, J.M., et al., Astrocyte-derived monocyte-chemoattractant protein-1 directs the transmigration of leukocytes across a model of the human blood-brain barrier. *J Immunol*, 1998. 161(12): p. 6896-903.

[77]Williams, K.C., et al., Antigen presentation by human fetal astrocytes with the cooperative effect of microglia or the microglial-derived cytokine IL-1. *J Neurosci*, 1995. 15(3 Pt 1): p. 1869-78.

[78]Wong, G.H., et al., Inducible expression of H-2 and Ia antigens on brain cells. *Nature*, 1984. 310(5979): p. 688-91.

[79]Xu, L., et al., Susceptibility to apoptosis varies with time in culture for murine neurons and astrocytes: changes in gene expression and activity. *Neurol Res*, 2004. 26(6): p. 632-43.

[80]Yenari, M.A., et al., Microglia Potentiate Damage to Blood-Brain Barrier Constituents. Improvement by Minocycline In Vivo and In Vitro. *Stroke*, 2006. 37: in press

[81]Zeinstra, E., N. Wilczak, and J. De Keyser, [3H]dihydroalprenolol binding to beta adrenergic receptors in multiple sclerosis brain. *Neurosci Lett*, 2000. 289(1): p. 75-7.

[82]Zeinstra, E., et al., Astrocytes in chronic active multiple sclerosis plaques express MHC class II molecules. *Neuroreport*, 2000. 11(1): p. 89-91.

[83]Zhang, Z.G., et al., Up-regulation of neuropilin-1 in neovasculature after focal cerebral ischemia in the adult rat. *J Cereb Blood Flow Metab*, 2001. 21(5): p. 541-9.

In: Inflammation Research Perspectives
Editor: Giacomo T. Romano, pp. 17-39
ISBN: 978-1-60021-845-3

Chapter II

Inflammation in Type 2 Diabetes and the Metabolic Syndrome

Ali A. Rizvi[*]
Division of Endocrinology, Diabetes, and Metabolism, University of South Carolina, School of Medicine, Columbia, SC 29203 USA

Abstract

The role of endothelial dysfunction and endovascular inflammation in the etiology of many disease states is in the process of being unravelled.The metabolic syndrome, type 2 diabetes, obesity, and related conditions have a common underlying pathophysiology of insulin resistance, vasculo-endothelial abnormalities, and a heightened proinflammatory state. A wealth of recent evidence shows that elevated levels of various inflammatory markers are associated with the presence and severity of these pathophysiologic processes, and may, to some extent, serve as mediators in a chronic atherosclerotic disease setting. C- reactive protein is the most extensively studied of these substances, but the list includes of postulated markers includes a whole host of other molecules like interleukin-1 and the adipocytokines. Investigation into their possible role in contributing to adverse clinical outcomes has generated intense excitement, making them targets of future therapeutic modalities. Improved understanding of these markers promises to enhance our efforts at prevention and treatment of these states of insulin resisitance.

[*] Correspondence concerning this article should be addressed to: Ali A. Rizvi, MD, FACP, Associate Professor of Medicine, Division of Endocrinology, Diabetes, and Metabolism, University of South Carolina School of Medicine, Two Medical Park, Suite 502, Columbia, SC 29203, USA. Ph: 803-540-1000; Fax: 803-540-1050; Email: arizvi@gw.mp.sc.edu.

Keywords: metabolic syndrome, inflammation, C-reactive protein, adipocytokines, insulin resistance.

Vascular Inflammation, Insulin Resistance and Atherosclerosis in the Metabolic Syndrome

There is currently an epidemic of type 2 diabetes and the metabolic syndrome because of enhanced rates of obesity, physical inactivity, and the ageing of the population, thus feuling the increase in cardiovascular diseases [1]. The metabolic syndrome, or "insulin resistance syndrome", consists of a clustering of cardiovascular risk factors in the setting of increased body weight (indicated mainly by increased waist circumference and body mass index or BMI). There is a significant overlap between the metabolic syndrome and type 2 diabetes. Is is thought that Insulin resistance is believed to play a major role in the underlying pathophysiology of these conditions, contributing to atherosclerosis and increasing the risk of cardiovascular events [2]. Thus a process of chronic and progressive damage to the arterial wall begins that eventually leads to atherosclerotic vascular complications. The resultant adverse sequelae are usually clinically evident and well recognized. The various stages of the atherosclerotic process have been delineated [3], and have their origins in insults to the endothelium from a combination of factors. These predisposing conditions include the well-known risk factors, including hypertension, hyperlipidemia, hyperglycemia, and smoking [4]. Sustained noxious stimuli interact over time to damage the vascular integrity and shift the balance of the endothelial milieu towards one that promotes injury and progressive failure of repair mechanisms [5]. Chemotaxis of mononuclear cells ensues, leading to their adhesion, migration, and differentiation within the vessel wall. Deposition of lipids within the macrophages is favored by the availability of easily oxidizable lipoproteins. Meanwhile, migration and proliferation of smooth muscle cells into the intima forms a fibrous cap over this "fatty streak" and leads to the appearance of an atherosclerotic lesion [6]. At some point during its subsequent progression, the altered pathology predisposes to the formation of a thrombus, usually initiated by plaque rupture. Indeed, vulnerable plaques have been identified that seem to have distinctive morphological composition and are prone to rupture [7]. The end-result is a vascular event that can have catastrophic consequences.

It is generally agreed that a heightened, proinflammatory picture precedes and perpetuates the atherosclerotic process [8]. Under healthy conditions, a delicate balance is maintained between the anti-inflammatory and pro-inflammatory forces acting on the endothelium (figure 1). The integrity of the endo-vasculature prevents the pro-atherogenic factors from predominating. However, there may be an increased genetic susceptibility to oxidative stress that lays the groundwork for ongoing damage [9]. Insulin resistance has been implicated in not only accelerating the inflammation [10], but also being the ultimate catalyst for glucose intolerance, dyslipidemia, and hypertensive damage. The picture, however, is complicated and controversial. The "insulin resistance hypothesis" contends that an inability to satisfactorily maintain insulin-mediated glucose uptake into tissues has a broad array of deleterious ramifications, some of which can be directly linked to the resultant hyperinsulinemia [11]. However, both the NCEP ATP III and the IDF criteria for the diagnosis of the metabolic syndrome are based on clinical and laboratory measurements and are devoid of the need for direct computation of insulin resistance [12,13]. What is established is the unequivocal importance of these criteria as risk factors for cardiovascular disease and type 2 diabetes. Therefore, the central role of insulin resistance in a definition of the metabolic syndrome meant for use in clinical practice is unclear. In addition, weight gain and obesity will increase both inflammation and insulin resistance [14]. In fact, in some studies, the bulk of association between the two can be explained on the basis of increased body weight alone [15]. However, not all obese individuals are insulin-resistant or display a proinflammatory picture. In short, although the metabolic syndrome had its origins as the "insulin resistance syndrome" and is still preferred to be called by that name by some people, the part that insulin resistance itself plays in its causation and sequelae is yet to be fully defined. On the other hand, a wealth of evidence is accumulating regarding the connection between markers of inflammation and the clinically-defined 'metabolic syndrome' [16,17].

Figure 1 – Factors affecting the integrity and function of the vascular endothelium

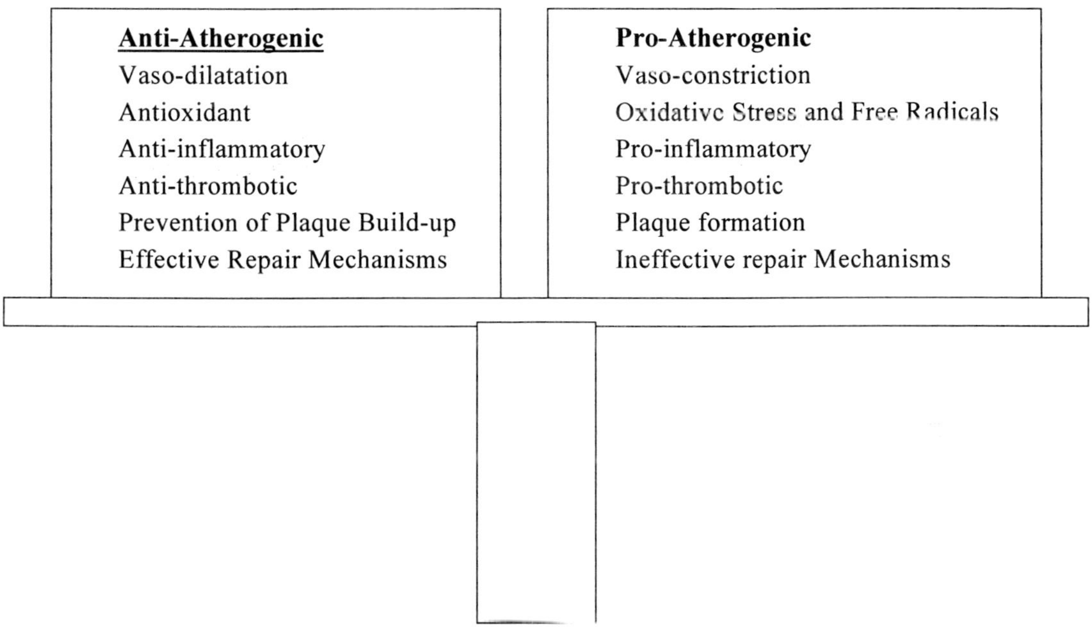

Inflammatory Markers as Emerging Risk Factors

Inflammation is regarded as a contributor to morbidity in the closely related conditions of cardiovascular disease, obesity, the metabolic syndrome, and type 2 diabetes and has been the focus of extensive research recently [18,19]. Inflammatory markers like C-reactive protein (CRP), fibrinogen, the interleukins, tumor necrosis factor-alpha (TNF-α), tissue-type plasminogen activator, and serum amyloid A (SAA) have been included in the ever-expanding list of emerging or "non-traditional" risk factors for the atherosclerotic process [20] (table 1). They mirror oxidative stress and generation of free radicals that can promote vascular damage, endothelial injury, plaque rupture, and athero-thrombosis [21]. Studies have established a significant inflammatory component in the background of clinically recognizable risk factors (for example, hypertension, hyperglycemia, dyslipidemia, obesity, and smoking) [22]. Inflammatory proteins like CRP have been shown to predict, and correlate independently with, major cardiovascular end-points like myocardial infarction and death [23,24]. The proposed interplay of the inflammatory mediators between the liver, fatty tissue, and the endothelium is shown in figure 2.

Table 1 – The Inflammatory Markers

Atherogenic
C - reactive protein
Interleukin-6
Tumor Necrosis Factor-α
Plasminogen Activator Inhibitor-1
Leptin
Resistin
Serum Amyloid A
Anti-atherogenic
Adiponectin

Hypercoagulability states and hemostatic factors like fibrinogen have been postulated to play a pathologic role in the development of vascular complications, ostensibly through abnormal rheology and elevated blood viscosity [25,26]. Prospective studies show that low-grade systemic inflammation is associated with not only the development of diabetes, but also its large-vessel and microvascular complications [27,28,29]. Retinopathy and nephropathy are linked to increased levels of inflammatory markers in both type 1 and type 2 diabetes [30,31]. However, it is not clear if CRP measurement in diabetes and the metabolic syndrome provides added information beyond that obtained through the established risk factors. Increased body mass index (BMI) with or without the presence of the metabolic syndrome or diabetes, accounted for the bulk of the pro-inflammatory picture in some analyses [28]. The effect of race on variation in inflammatory markers has also been noted in Caucasians and African-Americans [32]. Therefore, more research is needed before screening can be advocated [32,33].

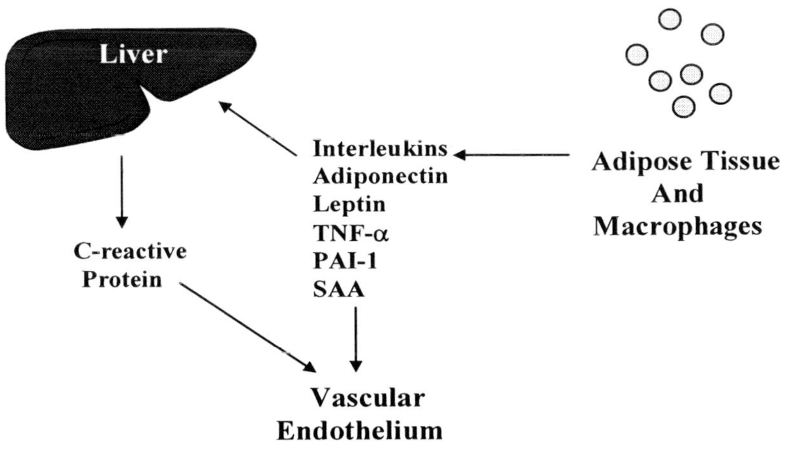

Figure 2. Interactions between adipose tissue, liver, and the vascular endothelium by way of the inflammatory markers and cytokines.

Since cardiovascular disease (CVD) and the metabolic syndrome are closely linked, any discussion of cardiac risk factors must necessarily overlap with the criteria designated for the metabolic syndrome. The traditional risk factors for CVD – positive family history, hypertension, diabetes, dyslipidemia, and smoking explain a preponderant amount of morbidity and mortality, especially when combined with abdominal obesity, sedentary lifestyle, and diet composition. However, these traditional or established factors do not fully account for the CVD burden in certain populations (for example, those with diabetes) [34,35]. Attention has been focused recently on whether the "nontraditional" risk factors are independently associated with vascular risk, and if they provide clinically significant prognostic value beyond the established ones [35,36]. Interestingly, these emerging factors are almost exclusively circulating markers, and tend to cluster together among themselves and with the traditional factors [37]. Examples of these markers that have been studied in some detail include CRP, fibrinogen, the adipocytokines, and the proinflammatory cytokines. Several epidemiologic studies demonstrate that CRP is a reliable predictor of future cardiovascular events in individuals free of disease at baseline [23,24]. However, three important questions remain to be answered in the analysis of these new risk factors vis-à-vis coronary disease: firstly, since these parameters are acute-phase reactants that segregate with the traditional risk factors, do they confer some measure of independent risk or merely reflect what can already be gleaned from known information? Second, are they simply markers or do they represent true mediators of the underlying extent of inflammation? Some argue that they are simply epiphenomena with little direct pathogenetic role in disease causation. However, the inherent proinflammatory actions of some of these markers point to a possible etiologic and pathologic implication in the disease process. Finally, it is not yet clear if clinical management can be altered on the basis of screening for these emerging factors. The answer to this last question is predicated on whether a treatment is developed that directly targets the various inflammatory markers without altering the established risk factors and subsequently evaluating clinical outcomes.

The Role of C-reactive Protein

CRP is the best-known marker of inflammation and has been touted as an independent risk factor for cardiovascular disease on the basis of recent studies. It is a member of the pentraxin family, which consists of five noncovalently associated peptides surrounding a central core. It is an acute-phase reactant that is synthesized in the liver and activates the classical pathway of complement through the immune system. Various proinflammatory cytokines such as tumor necrosis factor and interleukin-1 derived from vascular endothelium and adipose tissue stimulate its formation. The release of interleukin-6 from macrophages by increased oxidative stress and infection may be the original insult that initiates this process. CRP has been shown to tilt the balance of endovascular health towards a proatherogenic state by reducing the synthesis and biological activity of nitric oxide, upregulating endothelin-1, and activating cell adhesion molecules.

Numerous studies have revealed that persons that have the most or all features of the metabolic syndrome have increased levels of CRP [38,39,40]. It has been linked to insulin resistance, dyslipidemic states, blood pressure, and increased amounts of other proinflammatory cytokines [41]. The Insulin Resistance and Atherosclerosis Study showed that CRP values correlated with body mass index (BMI), waist circumference, and fasting hyperinsulinemia [42]. There is a linear correlation between CRP and the number of metabolic abnormalities present, namely upper-body obesity, dyslipidemia, hyperglycemic states, and hypertension [43]. For all levels of glucose, the presence of metabolic syndrome was associated with an increase in the prevalence of CVD [44]. The metabolic syndrome appears to be associated with inflammation in addition to being an important marker of CVD risk. CVD prevalence is greater in persons with metabolic syndrome without diabetes than in those with diabetes who do not have the metabolic syndrome [45]. CRP levels in nondiabetic persons increase with worsening glycemia and particularly with postload glycemia [46,47]. The Third National Health and Nutrition Examination Survey (NHANES III) data confirmed that subjects with the metabolic syndrome were more likely to have higher levels of CRP and other markers of inflammation [45]. Based on Framingham scores, CRP adds prognostic information to the predictive power of other CVD risk factors like cholesterol, hypertension, and cigarette use [20]. It confers a stronger predisposition to CVD than other known inflammatory markers such as homocysteine, IL-6, and SAA, circulating levels of which parallel CRP, intracellular adhesion molecule-1 (ICAM)-I [48,49], as well as low-density lipoprotein (LDL), the time-honored correlate of cardiovascular risk [50]. Obese persons have improvement in insulin sensitivity and in CRP with weight loss. On the other hand, obese persons with normal insulin sensitivity with low CRP levels do not show further decrease following weight loss. This suggests that improvement in insulin sensitivity rather than weight loss mediates the reduction in CRP levels [51]. Therefore, our understanding of the impact of various pathogenetic factors on CRP is still murky but in the process of being clarified (table 2).

Table 2 – Factors that affect circulating CRP levels

Increase in CRP
Obesity
Sedentary lifestyle
Acute infection
Trauma
Inflammatory disorders
Hyperglycemia
Decrease in CRP
Weight loss
Regular physical activity
Lipid-lowering (statin) therapy
Aspirin use

The reasons for the discrepant results regarding the benefit of using CRP in evaluating risk are not known. Possible explanations include different sets of populations studied, and their retrospective versus prospective nature. CRP, as well as other inflammatory markers, is acutely elevated in stress, illnesses, infections, and vascular events like myocardial infarction and unstable angina. CRP appears to be of greatest use in risk assessment of persons who have intermediate CVD risk (10-20%/10 years) [22]. Insulin resistance is associated with increased CRP levels, and in some studies CRP has been found to be an independent CVD risk factor [52-56]and a marker of insulin resistance [57-60]. Three studies examined the relationship between CRP, the metabolic syndrome, and incident cardiovascular events [57,61,62]. In these large population studies, CRP was a strong independent predictor of events, and its predictive value was equal to that of the metabolic syndrome. In two studies [55,61] the age-adjusted relative risk of future events was the same in subjects with high CRP without the metabolic syndrome and in subjects with low CRP with the metabolic syndrome. Interestingly, in subjects with both elevated CRP levels and the presence of the metabolic syndrome, the relative risk of events was double than in the other subgroups. This indicates that CRP measurement might have extra predictive power when added to the clinical definition of the metabolic syndrome. Rutter et al. [62] also found that CRP and the metabolic syndrome were independent risk factors, but in contrast to the two other reports, combining CRP and metabolic syndrome did not improve the predictive value of either used alone. Reilly et al. [63] also found that CRP did not add significantly to the metabolic syndrome, but their study did not include CVD outcomes.

Thus, there have been conflicting results when CRP has been used to evaluate risk of atherosclerotic vascular disease. It is possible that various types of populations have differing risks with respect to CRP. A retrospective, rather than prospective analysis may affect the conclusions as well. For instance, CRP is acutely elevated in stress, illnesses, infections, and vascular events like myocardial infarction and unstable angina. Various factors that affect CRP levels are summarized in table 2. An elevated CRP may simply signify an associative, rather than causative relationship with the endpoints being studied. It appears to be of greatest use in risk assessment of persons who have intermediate CVD risk (10-20%/10 years) (22).

The Adipocytokines

Our understanding of the functions of the adipose tissue has changed significantly with research suggesting that it not merely an inert storage site for excess energy. Instead, fatty tissue appears to be hormonally active and gives rise to a number of biologically active substances that regulate, and correlate with, insulin sensitivity, vascular function, and atherosclerotic disease. Collectively known as "adipocytokines", these molecules include, but are not limited to, adiponectin, leptin, resistin, IL-6, TNF-α, and plasminogen activator inhibitor-1 (PAI-1). An emerging concept is that obesity leads to infiltration of adipose tissues by macrophages which produce most of the inflammatory cytokines that are commonly measured [19] and contribute to insulin resistance. In addition, both macrophages and adipose tissue cells are thought to produce factors like IL-6 that secondarily increase hepatic CRP synthesis. Overfeeding may lead to a state of chronic macrophage activation, increased cytokines, central obesity, insulin resistance, and overproduction of the hepatic products of cytokine activation.

Adiponectin: The "Good" Cytokine

Adiponectin is produced by fat cells, and has properties that inhibit inflammation and enhance insulin sensitivity. It increases glucose transport and fatty acid oxidation. In animal studies, a deficiency of this cytokine can permit changes in metabolism to take place that favor the development of a metabolic syndrome phenotype [64]. It has been shown to suppress endothelial dysfunction, lipid accumulation, smooth muscle proliferation, and inhibit atherosclerotic changes in vessel walls. Low levels of adiponectin are found in subjects with diabetes and obesity, and correlate with insulin resistance and the future development of glucose intolerance and the metabolic syndrome. It has anti-inflammatory and antiatherogenic properties at the molecular level, such as decreasing the expression of adhesion molecules, reducing monocyte adhesion to endothelial cells, and suppressing various proatherogeic steps, such as uptake of oxidized LDL, foam cell formation, and proliferation and migration of vascular smooth muscle cells [65]. Other effects include increased insulin sensitivity and free fatty-acid oxidation oxidation, and decreased hepatic glucose production, and intracellular triglycerides. Adiponectin levels are lower in obesity and in prediabetes, and persons with higher levels of adiponectin have greater insulin sensitivity regardless of weight [66].

The question of whether a better understanding of the relationship between adiponectin and inflammation will lead to new or improved ways of addressing the metabolic syndrome is still unresolved. The connection between adiponectin and the clinical correlates of the metabolic syndrome is complex. It is interesting that obesity by itself in not necessarily associated with hypoleptinemia. Visceral obesity is predominantly associated with reduced levels of adiponectin. Obese women who have normal amounts of upper-body adipose tissue have normal adiponectin levels [67]. Low adiponectin was predictive of an increased future risk of coronary thrombosis in the Health Professionals Follow-up Study (HPFS), even after controlling for age, body weight, blood pressure, glucose control, physical activity, and tobacco use [68]. There seems to be a close relationship between adiponectin and HDL cholesterol [67,68] and the predictive power of adiponectin can partly be explained on their co-segregation.

In summary, adiponectin is inversely associated with insulin resistance, inflammation, blood pressure, LDL cholesterol, HDL cholesterol, and triglyceride levels. Multiple studies have established a correlation between adiponectin and CVD [69-72] and low levels of this adipocytokine found in subjects with the clinical characteristics of the metabolic syndrome. Uncontrolled hyperglycemia and diabetes is also associated with low levels of adiponectin [65].

THE PROINFLAMMATORY ADIPOCYTOKINES

The majority of adipocytokines correlate with positively with both insulin resistance and hyperinsulinemia in type 2 diabeets and the metabolic syndrome. Since they are also elevated in obesity and in the presence of cardiovascular risk factors [42], they provide further evidence towards the idea that inflammation is an integral part of the components of the metabolic syndrome. CRP, the most extensively studied inflammatory marker, is strongly associated with adipose-derived cytokines including interleukin-6 and TNF-α [73]. These are likely to be elevated in obese insulin-resistant subjects, especially in those with upper-body fat deposition, but not generally in obese subjects who are insulin-sensitive [51]. Since these markers have been linked to dyslipidemia, hypertension, and insulin levels [42,74], they have been implicated in the genesis and progression of CVD [7,17].

Interleukin-6 is a cytokine that is produced in part in the adipose tissue, especially omental fat. It is released in response to stress and stimulation through the sympathetic nervous system. Several studies suggest that it is a central mediator of the inflammatory response, and tends to correlates closely with CRP [75,76]. IL-6 is increased with increasing insulin resistance and in the presence of multiple features of the metabolic syndrome [77]. It increases hepatic triglyceride secretion and may be a factor in central obesity and insulin resistance. It seems to exert its metabolic actions both through its actions in the central nervous system (CNS) and on peripheral organs. Levels of IL-6 are linked to insulin resistance and adiposity [78]. Its exact pathogenetic in glucose and lipid homeostasis in human is still a matter of debate.

Tumor Necrosis Factor-α is produced by largely by adipose tissue, but also by macrophages and endothelial cells. Its levels correlate with amount of adipose tissue, and it has a role in modulating insulin sensitivity [79]. It has been linked to the increase in insulin resistance seen with obesity [80], although a consistent correlation of TNF-α with BMI has not been conclusively demonstrated. Although it has been implicated in states of increased insulin resistance, passive immunization with antibodies to TNF-α does not improve insulin sensitivity.

The discovery of *leptin* generated great interest when it was found to have a role in obesity, energy balance, and appetite regulation. Hypoleptinemia has been linked to weight gain, fat deposition in organs such as the liver, muscle, and pancreatic islets, clinical features of the metabolic syndrome, and a general proinflammatory state [81]. Leptin could have the property of lowering insulin levels. Resistance to leptin may be connected to the hyperinsulinemia that is the earliest compensatory defect in the pathway towards the metabolic syndrome and glucose intolerance. Efforts at harnessing the known properties of this hormone to therapeutic purposes have so far been unsuccessful.

Leptin is secreted by adipocytes and binds to receptors in the CNS, where it suppresses appetite and decreases food intake. In the peripheral tissues, it enhances insulin sensitivity in muscle and fatty tissue, while preventing fat storage in organs such as the liver and pancreas [82]. It functions as a signaling factor that keeps the CNS informed of the status of energy availability in the body, especially as it pertains to the adipose tissue. Weight gain and overfeeding increase leptin expression and secretion, while reduced food intake suppresses them [83]. Leptin deficient mice (*ob/ob* mice) manifest extreme obesity. In humans, typical obesity is associated with increased leptin levels, signifying underlying leptin resistance. Whether leptin-resistant individuals are, therefore, prone to becoming overweight or if obesity aggravates resistance to leptin action is not entirely clear. The metabolic syndrome is also associated with increased levels of leptin [84]. However, most of this elevation can probably be explained on the basis of the extra weight alone. Does insulin resistance and the presence of other features of the metabolic syndrome modulate leptin release, or are more apt to be present if leptin resistance is present, is the subject of future debate and research.

Additional research has unveiled another adipocyte-derived cytokine, *resistin,* that is elevated in obesity and impaired glucose tolerance. Its role in the genesis and pathophysiology of the metabolic syndrome, however, remains to be fully elucidated.

Other Inflammatory Markers

Insulin resistance is associated with a number of other inflammatory markers that have generated interest, such as secretory phospholipase A2, e-selectin, ICAM-1, and SAA [17]. Most of these are acute-phase reactants, whose production in the liver is induced by the interleukins and TNF-α. SAA appears to be a "scavenger" apolipoprotein that is closely linked with high-density lipoprotein (HDL). t is involved in lipid transport in the circulation, accelerating cholesterol uptake from damaged tissues, and may also play a role in immune regulation. Increased levels SAA that are seen after myocardial infarction are associated with an elevated risk of a recurrent coronary event [84]. In short, it may have an integrative role in such seemingly diverse areas as inflammation, atherosclerosis, and immunity. Further research is essential to unraveling its exact place in the inflammatory cascade and the obesity-metabolic syndrome spectrum. It is safe to say that, based on results of research done thus far, the inflammatory cytokines are critical in affecting the balance of endothelial health;

obesity, insulin resistance, stress, presence of the metabolic syndrome components, and other acute or chronic insults tend to tilt the balance towards a more proinflammatory picture and lead an environment conducive to atherogenesis and thrombosis. Components of the metabolic syndrome as well as the syndrome itself are associated with various measures of inflammation. This inflammatory picture is low-grade but chronic, and is associated with an increased risk for cardiovascular disease and diabetes. It provides a putative pathogenetic mechanism for the increased risk of adverse vascular outcomes that are experienced by individuals with the metabolic syndrome.

HYPERCOAGULABLITY AND HEMOSTASIS

The metabolic syndrome and type 2 diabetes have been found to be associated with increased levels of fibrinogen [85,86] enhanced platelet adhesion [87] and impaired fibrinolysis [88,89] and elevated PAI-1 [90]. The latter is probably the most consistent abnormality seen in persons with the metabolic syndrome. In addition, endothelial dysfunction is linked to increased levels of clotting factors like factor VIII and von Willibrand's factor [91]. These changes are closely associated with insulin resistance and cardiovascular risk factors. The overall effect is an increased tendency to clotting and thrombus formation, as well as a reduced capacity to mitigate the pro-thrombotic tendency from impaired fibrinolysis. An elevated risk of atherothrombosis and cardiovascular obstructive events ensues.

PAI-1 levels are strongly associated with dyslipidemia, hyperinsulinemia, and hypertension [92,93]. It is noteworthy that the effect of increased PAI-1 was mitigated to a nonsignificant level after adjusting for BMI and elevated triglycerides in one study [94] In the Cardiovascular Health Study [93] levels of procoagulant factors and vitamin K-dependent proteins were studied in association with the different components of the metabolic syndrome. PAI-1 stood out as having the most consistent correlation with body weight, hyperglycemia, and hyperinsulinemia. TNF-α and IL-6 have been shown to induce synthesis of fibrinogen in the liver. Additional evidence of the connection between insulin resistance and defective fibrinolysis is provided by the possible involvement of the renin-angiotensin system and abnormalities of platelet function. The former is activated in obese, insulin-resistant subjects, who have higher levels of angiotensinogen and increased PAI-1 formation and release. Increased platelet activation and aggregation is found in subjects with the metabolic syndrome and type 2 diabetes as well [87].

Similarly, type 2 diabetes is considered to increase the risk of thrombosis, especially when present in conjunction with the metabolic syndrome [90]. Hypercoagulability and hemostatic factors like fibrinogen have been postulated to play a pathologic role in the development of diabetic complications, ostensibly through abnormal rheology and elevated blood viscosity [95] Elevated fibrinogen may offer a clue to the propensity to microvascular complications in patients with diabetes. Increased platelet activation and aggregation is found in subjects with type 2 diabetes as well [96].

In summary, the metabolic syndrome-type 2 diabetes spectrum is a hypercoagulable state that is a feature of the underlying insulin resistance that is common to both conditions. It predisposes to clot formation in the milieu of endothelial dysfunction, endovascular atheromatous change, and abnormal blood rheology. Studies to date have shown evidence for a pathophysiologic role of the inflammatory markers in promoting a prothrombotic tendency and impairing the ability of fibrinolytic repair and resumption of blood flow. However, many of the interconnections between the coagulation system, inflammation, and the individual risk factors of the metabolic syndrome have yet to be clearly delineated.

INFLAMMATORY MARKERS IN CHILDREN WITH THE METABOLIC SYNDROME AND OBESITY

The prevalence of obesity, the metabolic syndrome, and type 2 diabetes in the pediatric population is increasing at an exponential pace [97] [98]. Although a wealth of information about the metabolic syndrome has accumulated in adults, research about the prevalence and manifestations of the syndrome among children and adolescents is limited. Preliminary studies reveal that, like their adult counterparts, children and adolescents with the metabolic syndrome are more likely than those without this syndrome to show evidence of low-grade inflammation and increased levels of proinflammatory cytokines [98].

The association between obesity and elevated concentrations of CRP in children and adolescents has been clearly established [99,100]. The percentage of children and adolescents with an elevated concentration of CRP (>3.0 mg/l) is manifold higher among those with the metabolic syndrome compared with those who did not have the syndrome. In these studies, visceral obesity was the component that was responsible for much of the difference in concentrations of CRP. Concentrations of CRP have also been significantly associated with the other four components of the metabolic syndrome [101,102]. However, after adjustment for an anthropometric measure, many of these associations were seriously weakened and often failed to achieve statistical significance.

Although no studies have thus far shown that children and adolescents with evidence of low-grade inflammation are more likely to develop cardiovascular disease or diabetes than those without such evidence, obesity in childhood does increase the risk for diabetes in childhood and a variety of diseases in adulthood [103]. Results of a recent study suggest that the presence of the metabolic syndrome and abdominal obesity among children and adolescents may be lay the foundation for the emergence of cardiovascular disease and diabetes later in life through early low-grade inflammation [104]. To reduce the potential adverse effects of the inflammation that accompanies the metabolic syndrome, a concerted public health and behavioral approach is needed to reduce the burden of obesity and physical inactivity in children. Success in this endeavor will require a collaborative and multidisciplinary approach involving parents, school systems, state and government agencies, and professional organizations. This strategy will not only prevent the development of the syndrome and its attendant proinflammatory manifestations, but also ameliorate these features in those who already have the metabolic syndrome or its components

Effect of Various Interventions on Inflammatory Markers in the Metabolic Syndrome

The trio of the metabolic syndrome, cardiovascular disease, and increased inflammation has assumed enhanced priority because of their direct implication in fueling the epidemics of type 2 diabetes and vascular disease [17,105]. In the absence of any approved drug therapy, modulation of the inflammatory state by lifestyle factors in the metabolic syndrome assumes paramount importance [106]. This is even more significant in view of the fact that dietary factors and lack of physical activity in the modern-day world forms the basis for the enormous increase in the prevalence of the metabolic syndrome. It makes sense, therefore, to attack the very dynamics that contribute to the genesis of the syndrome. Attainment of an ideal body weight and normalization of BMI, preferably by a combination of physical activity and a calorie-restricted diet, form the cornerstone of therapeutic measures for the metabolic syndrome. Weight loss has been shown to reduce the inflammatory markers associated with insulin resistance. The composition of the diet is important as well – a Mediterranean-style diet rich in fruits, nuts, whole grains, and olive oil has been shown to have a beneficial effect on the metabolic syndrome and its clinical and inflammatory components [107]. Polyunsaturated, omega-3, and linoleic acid supplementation has also been shown to help [108]. Weight loss reduces the prevalence of steatohepatitis, an emerging facet of the metabolic syndrome that is closely associated with increased inflammatory markers [109]. Exercise has been shown to reduce the proinfammatory and prothrombotic picture in individuals who have the clinical criteria of the metabolic syndrome [110]. Sustained physical activity also has a salutary effect on chemokines and other mediators in insulin resistance [111]. The involvement of dieticians and other health care professionals is of vital importance in educating individuals of the need for dietary modifications in preventing the adverse sequelae of obesity and the metabolic syndrome [112]. Cigarette smoking has been shown to elevate proinflammatory markers as well as insulin resistance itself in a Japanese study [113].

There are no drugs that have been approved solely for the treatment of the metabolic syndrome or for targeting the heightened inflammatory state involved therein. At the time of writing, no guidelines recommend routine testing, targeting, or monitoring of CRP levels, the most extensively studies marker in states on insulin resistance. However, medication already in use for the treatment of metabolic conditions like diabetes, hypertension, and dyslipidemia have been shown to reduce inflammation in susceptible individuals through various mechanisms. A detailed description of the actions of these drugs on markers of inflammation is beyond the scope of this review. Perhaps the best known are the thiazolidinediaones, agents that directly ameliorate insulin resistance by acting on the peroxisome-proliferator activator receptor-gamma (PPAR-γ) nuclear receptors. Numerous studies have proven their efficacy in reducing markers of inflammation [114,115,116] and improving endothelial function and lipid profile and blood pressure. The two agents currently available on the market, rosiglitazone and pioglitazone, have both been studied in this respect. An unwanted side-effect, however, is the tendency to weight gain, fluid accumulation, and possible precipitation of overt congestive heart failure. Although this class of medications is widely used for the treatment of type 2 diabetes, it is not yet approved for use in prediabetes or the metabolic syndrome.

Several other medications have approved indications and target risk factors for cardiovascular disease as well as individual components of the metabolic syndrome. The HMG Co-A reductase inhibitors ("statins") are proven for their lipid-lowering properties and for reducing cardiac and all-cause mortality. Several large clinical trials showed that they decreased inflammatory markers, notably CRP levels, in high-risk individuals with dyslipidemia, diabetes, and the metabolic syndrome [55,117,118]. This action is part of their non-lipid-lowering, or pleotropic, efficacy on the vascular endothelium [119,120]. Fibric-acid derivatives have also been advocated as useful agents in counter-acting the elevated inflammatory milieu of the metabolic syndrome [121].

Two other therapeutic modalities appear to be beneficial in the metabolic syndrome by reducing the proinflammatory and thrombotic cascade: targeting the renin-angiotensin system through the use of angiotensin-converting enzyme inhibitors [122] and angiotensin-receptor blocking agents [123] and use of aspirin to decrease the primary as well as secondary incidence of coronary thrombosis in patients with existing cardiovascular disease or those with multiple risk factors [124]. Most individuals with the metabolic syndrome will satisfy the clinical requirement for use of these agents and it is plausible that a significant portion of their salutary mechanisms are mediated by means of their anti-inflammatory actions. Specifically targeting the inflammatory pathways and mediators in insulin resistance and the metabolic syndrome is still uncharted territory, though a promising next step, of future drug therapy [125,126].

The Inflammatory Markers for Screening and as Therapeutic Targets

There is currently no consensus in using the markers of inflammation as screening tools or as risk factors to be targeted. This area appears to be embroiled in controversy and confusion, although some recommendations have been put forth [8,9]. The argument for testing of individuals at moderate risk for cardiovascular disease is based on further stratifying their risk status and assist in clinical management. On the other hand, some contend that the role of these acute-phase reactants in disease causation is not established, and therefore screening would not be helpful in leading to a change in management strategy for the majority of patients tested. Additionally, the lack of specific and proven therapeutic interventions targeting these markers (beyond what is already being recommended) is also a factor against using them in routine clinical setting. Whether to include CRP or some other inflammatory marker in the clinical criteria used in the diagnosis of the metabolic syndrome is dependent upon elucidation of their exact role in the pathogenesis of the syndrome and their connection to underlying insulin resistance. In other words, the question of whether these markers are merely the mirror of a chronic vasculotoxic pattern or are causally involved in endothelial dysfunction and atherosclerosis is central from the viewpoint of using them for screening, assessment, and treatment in the metabolic syndrome and related conditions. Further research is needed to clarify the etiology of the metabolic syndrome at the molecular and inflammatory level and possibly to a definition that includes one or more of the inflammatory markers. Hopefully, a new model of the metabolic syndrome can be validated so that its predictive value is inclusive of clinical as well as laboratory criteria. Additional studies concerning the markers of inflammation, ideally performed in a prospective, randomized, and interventional manner, should help in translating the knowledge gained in the laboratory to the bedside.

The Inflammatory Markers and Endothelial Health: Conclusion

Relevant research suggests that the inflammatory cytokines discussed above are critical in affecting the balance of endothelial health. Obesity, insulin resistance, stress, presence of the metabolic syndrome components, hyperglycemia, and other acute or chronic insults tend to tilt the balance towards a more proinflammatory picture and lead an environment conducive to atherogenesis and thrombosis. This inflammatory picture is low-grade but chronic, is associated with an increased risk for cardiovascular disease, and provides a possible pathogenetic mechanism for the increased risk of adverse vascular outcomes that are experienced by individuals with the metabolic syndrome and diabetes.

References

[1] Grundy SM. Obesity, metabolic syndrome, and cardiovascular disease. *J Clin Endocrinol Metab* 2004;89(6):2595-2600.

[2] Reaven GM. Insulin resistance, cardiovascular disease, and the metabolic syndrome: how well do the emperor's clothes fit? *Diabetes Care* 2004;27:1011-1012.

[3] Ross R: Atherosclerosis: an inflammatory disease. *N. Engl. J. Med.* 1999;340:115–126.

[4] Wannamethee SG, Lowe GD, Shaper AG, Rumley A, Lennon L, Whiner PH, Insulin resistance, haemostatic and inflammatory markers and coronary heart disease risk factors in type 2 diabetic men with and without coronary heart disease. *Diabetologia.* 2004;47(9):1557-1565.

[5] Sjoholm A, Nystrom T. Endothelial inflammation in insulin resistance. *Lancet* 2005;365(9459):610-612.

[6] Ceriello A, Motz E. Is oxidative stress the pathogenic mechanism underlying insulin resistance, diabetes, and cardiovascular disease? The common soil hypothesis revisited. *Arterioscler. Thromb. Vasc. Biol.* 2004;24:816-823.

[7] Hansson JK. Inflammation, atherosclerosis, and coronary artery disease. *N. Engl. J. Med.* 2005;352:1685-1695.

[8] Black PH. The inflammatory response is an integral part of the stress response: Implications for atherosclerosis, insulin resistance, type II diabetes and metabolic syndrome X. *Brain. Behav. Immun.* 2003 Oct;17(5):350-64. Review.

[9] Shinozaki K, Kashiwagi A, Masada M, Okamura T. Molecular mechanisms of impaired endothelial function associated with insulin resistance. *Curr. Drug. Targets Cardiovasc. Haematol. Disord.* 2004;4:1-11.

[10] Fernandez-Real JM, Ricart W. Insulin resistance and chronic cardiovascular inflammatory syndrome. *Endocr. Rev.* 2003;24(3):278-301.

[11] Reaven GM, Laws A. Insulin resistance, compensatory hyperinsulinaemia, and coronary heart disease. *Diabetologia.* 1994;37(9):948-52.

[12] Expert Panel on Detection, Evaluation, and Treatment of High Blood Cholesterol in Adults: Executive Summary of the Third Report of the National Cholesterol Education Program (NCEP) Expert Panel on Detection, Evaluation, and Treatment of High Blood Cholesterol in Adults (Adult Treatment Panel III). *JAMA*, 2001;285:2486-2497.

[13] International Diabetes Federation: The IDF consensus worldwide definition of the metabolic syndrome. IDF Executive Office, Brussels, Belgium. *www.idf.org.*

[14] Clinical guidelines on the Identification, Evaluation, and Treatment of Overweight and Obesity in Adults – The Evidence Report, National Institutes of Health. *Obes. Res.* 1998;6(suppl 2):51S-209S.

[15] Sung RY, Tong PC, YU CW, et al. High prevalence of insulin reistance and metabolic syndrome in overweight/obese preadolescent Homg Kong Chinese children aged 9-12 years. *Diabetes Care* 2003;26:250-151.

[16] Chan JC, Cheung JC, Stehouwer CD, Emeis JJ, Tong PC, Ko GT, Yudkin JS. The central roles of obesity-associated dyslipidaemia, endothelial activation and cytokines in the Metabolic Syndrome--an analysis by structural equation modelling. *Int. J. Obes. Relat. Metab. Disord.* 2002;26(7):994-1008.

[17] Tracy RP. Inflammation, the metabolic syndrome and cardiovascular risk. *Int. J. Clin. Pract. Suppl.* 2003;134:10-17.

[18] Danesh J, Wheeler JG, Hirschfield GM, et al. C-reactive protein and other markers of inflammation in the prediction of coronary artery disease. *N. Engl. J. Med.* 2004;350:1387-1397.

[19] Wannamethee SG, Lowe GD, Shaper AG, Rumley A, Lennon L, Whiner PH, Insulin resistance, haemostatic and inflammatory markers and coronary heart disease risk factors in type 2 diabetic men with and without coronary heart disease. *Diabetalogia* 2004;47(9):1557-1565.

[20] Muntner P, He J, Chen J, Fonseca V, Whelton PK. Prevalence of non-traditional cardiovascular risk factors among persons with impaired fasting glucose, impaired glucose tolerance, diabetes, and the metabolic syndrome: analysis of the Third National Health and Nutrition Examination Survey (NHANES III). *Ann. Epidemiol.* 2004;14(9):686-695.

[21] Hsueh WA, Quinones MJ. Role of endothelial dysfunction in insulin resistance. *Am. J. Cardiol.* 2003:92:10J-17J.

[22] Pearson TA, Mensah GA, Alexander RW, et al. Markers of inflammation and cardiovascular disease: application to clinical and public health practice: a statement for healthcare professionals from the Centers for Disease Control and Prevention and the American Heart Association. *Circulation* 2003;107:499-511.

[23] Ridker PM, Cushman M, Stampfer MJ, Tracy RP, Hennekens CH. Inflammation, aspirin, and the risk of cardiovascular disease in apparently healthy men. *N. Engl. J. Med.* 1997;336:973-979. (*Erratum, N. Engl. J. Med.* 1997;337:356).

[24] Ridker PM, Rifai N, Rose L, Buring JE, Cook NR. Comparison of C-reactive protein and low-density lipoprotein cholesterol levels in the prediction of first cardiovascular events. *N. Engl. J. Med.* 2002;347-1557-1565.

[25] Bruno G, Cavallo-Perin P, Bargero G, et al. Hyperfibrinogenemia and metabolic syndrome in type 2 diabetes: a population-based study. *Diabetes. Metab. Res. Rev.* 2001;17(2): 124-130.

[26] Carr ME. Diabetes mellitus: a hypercoagulable state. *J. Diabetes. Complications.* 2001;15(1):44-54.

[27] Stehouwer CDA, Gall M, Twisk JWR, Knudsen E, Emeis JJ, Parving H. Increased urinary albumin excretion, endothelial dysfunction, and chronic low-grade inflammation in type 2 diabetes. Progressive, interrelated, and independently associated with risk of death. *Diabetes* 2002;51:1157-1165.

[28] Duncan BB, Schmidt MI, Pankow JI, et al. Low-grade systemic inflammation and the development of type 2 diabetes. The Atherosclerosis Risk in Communities study. *Diabetes* 2003;52:1799-1805.

[29] Freeman DJ, Norrie J, Caslake MJ, et al. C-reactive protein is an independent predictor of risk for the development of diabetes in the West of Scotland Coronary Prevention Study. *Diabetes* 2002;51:1596-1600.

[30] Asakawa H, Tokunaga K, Kawakami F. Elevation of fibrinogen and thrombin-antithrombin III complex levels of type 2 diabetes patients with retinopathy and nephropathy. *J. Diabetes. Complications.* 2000;14(3):121-126.

[31] Saraheimo M, Teppo AM, Forsblom C, Fagerudd J, Groop PH. Diabetic nephropathy is associated with low-grade inflammation in type 1 diabetic patients. *Diabetalogia* 2003;46(10):1402-1407.

[32] Tall AR. C-reactive protein reassessed. *N Engl J Med* 2004;350:1450-1452.

[33] Mosca L. C-reactive protein – to screen or not to screen? *N. Engl. J. Med.* 2002;347:1615-1617.

[34] Hackam DG, Anand SS. Emerging risk factors for atherosclerotic vascular disease: a critical review of the evidence. *JAMA* 2003;290(7):932-940.

[35] Streja D, Cressey P, Rabkin SW. Associations between inflammatory markers, traditional risk factors, and complications in patients with type 2 diabetes mellitus. *J. Diabetes Complications* 2003;17(3):120-127.

[36] Bhatt DL, Topol EJ. Need to test the inflammation hypothesis. *Circulation* 2002;106:136-140.

[37] Ceriello A, Motz E. Is oxidative stress the pathogenic mechanism underlying insulin resistance, diabetes, and cardiovascular disease? The common soil hypothesis revisited. *Arterioscler. Thromb. Vasc. Biol.* 2004;24:816-823.

[38] Ridker PM, Buring JE, Cook NR, Rifai N. C-reactive protein, the metabolic syndrome, and risk of incident cardiovascular events: an 8-year follow-up of 14,719 initially healthy American women. *Circulation* 2003;107:391–397.

[39] Pradhan AD, Cook NR, Buring JE, Manson JE, Ridker PM. C-reactive protein is independently associated with fasting insulin in nondiabetic women. *Arterioscler. Thromb. Vasc. Biol.* 2003;23:650–655.

[40] Rutter MK, Meigs JB, Sullivan LM, D'Agostino RB Sr, Wilson PW. C-reactive protein, the metabolic syndrome, and prediction of cardiovascular events in the Framingham Offspring Study. *Circulation* 2004;110:380–385.

[41] Yudkin JS, Stehouwer CD, Emeis JJ, Coppack SW. C-reactive protein in healthy subjects: associations with obesity, insulin resistance, and endothelial dysfunction: a potential role for cytokines originating from adipose tissue? *Arterioscler. Thromb. Vasc. Biol.* 1999;19:972–978.

[42] Festa A, D'Agostino R Jr, Howard G, Mykkanen L, Tracy RP, Haffner SM. Chronic subclinical inflammation as part of the insulin resistance syndrome: the Insulin Resistance Atherosclerosis Study (IRAS). *Circulation* 102:42–47, 2000

[43] Ridker PM, Wilson PW, Grundy SM. Should C-reactive protein be added to metabolic syndrome and to assessment of global cardiovascular risk? *Circulation* 2004;109:2818–2825.

[44] Isomaa B, Almgren P, Tuomi T, Forsen B, Lahti K, Nissen M, Taskinen MR, Groop L. Cardiovascular morbidity and mortality associated with the metabolic syndrome. *Diabetes Care* 2001;24:683-689.

[45] Alexander CM, Landsman PB, Teutsch SM, Haffner SM, Third National Health and Nutrition Examination Survey (NHANES III), National Cholesterol Education Program (NCEP): NCEP-defined metabolic syndrome, diabetes, and prevalence of coronary heart disease among NHANES III participants age 50 years and older. *Diabetes* 2003;52:1210-1214.

[46] Freeman DJ, Norrie J, Caslake MJ, et al. C-reactive protein is an independent predictor of risk for the development of diabetes in the West of Scotland Coronary Prevention Study. *Diabetes* 2002;51:1596-1600.

[47] Pradhan A, Manson J, Rifai N, Buring J, Ridker P. C-reactive protein, interleukin 6, and risk of developing type 2 diabetes mellitus. *JAMA* 2001;286:3327-334.

[48] Hackam DG, Anand SS. Emerging risk factors for atherosclerotic vascular disease: a critical review of the evidence. *JAMA* 2003;290(7):932-940.

[49] Danesh J, Wheeler JG, Hirschfield GM, Eda S, Eiriksdottir G, Rumley A, Lowe GD, Pepys MB, Gudnason V: C-reactive protein and other circulating markers of inflammation in the prediction of coronary heart disease. *N. Engl. J. Med.* 2004;350: 1387-1397.

[50] Ridker PM, Rifai N, Rose L, Buring JE, Cook NR: Comparison of C-reactive protein and low-density lipoprotein cholesterol levels in the prediction of first cardiovascular events. *N. Engl. J. Med.* 2002;347: 1557-1565.

[51] McLaughlin T, Abbasi F, Lamendola C, Liang L, Reaven G, Schaaf P, Reaven P: Differentiation between obesity and insulin resistance in the association with C-reactive protein. *Circulation* 2002;106:2908-2912.

[52] Danesh J, Collins R, Appleby P, Peto R. Association of fibrinogen, C-reactive protein, albumin, or leukocyte count with coronary heart disease: meta-analyses of prospective studies. *JAMA* 1998;279:1477–1482.

[53] Ridker PM, Hennekens CH, Buring JE, Rifai N. C-reactive protein and other markers of inflammation in the prediction of cardiovascular disease in women. *N. Engl. J. Med.* 2000;342:836–843.

[54] Ridker PM. Clinical applications of C-reactive protein for cardiovascular disease detection and prevention. *Circulation* 2003;107:363–369.

[55] Ridker PM, Cannon CP, Morrow D, Rifai N, Rose LM, McCabe CH, Pfeffer MA, Braunwald E. C-reactive protein levels and outcomes after statin therapy: Pravastatin or Atorvastatin Evaluation and Infection Therapy-Thrombolysis in Myocardial Infarction 22 (PROVE IT-TIMI 22). *N. Engl. J. Med.* 2005;352:20–28.

[56] Ridker PM, Buring JE, Cook NR, Rifai N. C-reactive protein, the metabolic syndrome, and risk of incident cardiovascular events: an 8-year follow-up of 14,719 initially healthy American women. *Circulation* 2003;107:391–397.

[57] Pradhan AD, Cook NR, Buring JE, Manson JE, Ridker PM. C-reactive protein is independently associated with fasting insulin in nondiabetic women. *Arterioscler. Thromb. Vasc. Biol.* 2003;23:650–655.

[58] Yudkin JS, Stehouwer CD, Emeis JJ, Coppack SW. C-reactive protein in healthy subjects: associations with obesity, insulin resistance, and endothelial dysfunction: a potential role for cytokines originating from adipose tissue? *Arterioscler. Thromb. Vasc Biol.* 1999;19:972–978.

[59] McLaughlin T, Abbasi F, Lamendola C, Liang L, Reaven G, Schaaf P, Reaven P. Differentiation between obesity and insulin resistance in the association with C-reactive protein. *Circulation* 2002;106:2908–2912.

[60] Festa A, D'Agostino R Jr, Howard G, Mykkanen L, Tracy RP, Haffner SM. Chronic subclinical inflammation as part of the insulin resistance syndrome: the Insulin Resistance Atherosclerosis Study (IRAS). *Circulation* 2000;102:42–47.

[61] Sattar N, Gaw A, Scherbakova O, Ford I, O'Reilly DS, Haffner SM, Isles C, Macfarlane PW, Packard CJ, Cobbe SM, Shepherd J. Metabolic syndrome with and without C-reactive protein as a predictor of coronary heart disease and diabetes in the West of Scotland Coronary Prevention Study. *Circulation* 2003;108:414–419.

[62] Rutter MK, Meigs JB, Sullivan LM, D'Agostino RB Sr, Wilson PW. C-reactive protein, the metabolic syndrome, and prediction of cardiovascular events in the Framingham Offspring Study. *Circulation* 2004;110:380–385.

[63] Reilly MP, Wolfe ML, Rhodes T, Girman C, Mehta N, Rader DJ. Measures of insulin resistance add incremental value to the clinical diagnosis of metabolic syndrome in association with coronary atherosclerosis. *Circulation* 2004;110:803–809.

[64] Trujillo ME, Scherer PE. Adiponectin – journey from an adipocyte secretory protein to biomarker of the metabolic syndrome. *J. Intern. Med* .2005;257(2):167-175.

[65] Chandran M, Phillips SA, Ciaraldi T, Henry RR. Adiponectin: more than just another fat cell hormone? *Diabetes Care* 2003;26:2442–2450.

[66] Weyer C, Funahashi T, Tanaka S, Hotta K, Matsuzawa Y, Pratley RE, Tataranni PA. Hypoadiponectinemia in obesity and type 2 diabetes: close association with insulin resistance and hyperinsulinemia. *J. Clin. Endocrinol. Metab* .2001;86:1930–1935.

[67] Matsubara M, Maruoka S, Katayose S. Decreased plasma adiponectin concentrations in women with dyslipidemia. *J. Clin. Endocrinol. Metab.* 2002;87:2764–2769.

[68] Kazumi T, Kawaguchi A, Sakai K, Hirano T, Yoshino G. Young men with high-normal blood pressure have lower serum adiponectin, smaller LDL size, and higher elevated heart rate than those with optimal blood pressure. *Diabetes Care* 2002;25:971–976.

[69] Kumada M, Kihara S, Sumitsuji S, Kawamoto T, Matsumoto S, Ouchi N, Arita Y, Okamoto Y, Shimomura I, Hiraoka H, Nakamura T, Funahashi T, Matsuzawa Y, Osaka CAD Study Group. Association of hypoadiponectinemia with coronary artery disease in men. *Arterioscler. Thromb. Vasc. Biol.* 2003;23:85–89.

[70] Kojima S, Funahashi T, Sakamoto T, Miyamoto S, Soejima H, Hokamaki J, Kajiwara I, Sugiyama S, Yoshimura M, Fujimoto K, Miyao Y, Suefuji H, Kitagawa A, Ouchi N, Kihara S, Matsuzawa Y, Ogawa H. The variation of plasma concentrations of a novel, adipocyte derived protein, adiponectin, in patients with acute myocardial infarction. *Heart* 2003;89:667–672.

[71] Zoccali C, Mallamaci F, Tripepi G, Benedetto FA, Cutrupi S, Parlongo S, Malatino LS, Bonanno G, Seminara G, Rapisarda F, Fatuzzo P, Buemi M, Nicocia G, Tanaka S, Ouchi N, Kihara S, Funahashi T, Matsuzawa Y. Adiponectin, metabolic risk factors, and cardiovascular events among patients with end-stage renal disease. *J. Am. Soc. Nephrol.* 2002;13:134–141.

[72] Pischon T, Girman CJ, Hotamisligil GS, Rifai N, Hu FB, Rimm EB. Plasma adiponectin levels and risk of myocardial infarction in men. *JAMA* 2004;291:1730–1737.

[73] Kershaw EE, Flier JS: Adipose tissue as an endocrine organ. *J. Clin. Endocrinol. Metab.* 2004;89:2548–2556.

[74] Yudkin JS, Stehouwer CD, Emeis JJ, Coppack SW. C-reactive protein in healthy subjects: associations with obesity, insulin resistance, and endothelial dysfunction: a potential role for cytokines originating from adipose tissue? *Arterioscler. Thromb. Vasc Biol* 1999;19:972–978.

[75] McCarty MF. Interleukin-6 as a central mediator of cardiovascular risk associated with chronic inflammation, smoking, diabetes, and visceral obesity: down-regulation with essential fatty acids, ethanol, and pentoxifylline. *Med. Hypotheses*. 1999;52(5):465-477.

[76] Fasshauer M, Paschke R. Regulation of adipocytokines and insulin resistance. *Diabetologia* 2003;46(12):1594-1603.

[77] Vozarova B, Weyer C, Hanson K, et al. Circulating interleukin-6in relation to adiposity, insulin action, and insulin secretion. *Obes. Res.* 2001:9:414-417.

[78] Bastard JP, Jardel C, Bruckert E, Blondy P, Capeau J, Laville M, Vidal H, Hainque B. Elevated levels of interleukin 6 are reduced in serum and subcutaneous adipose tissue of obese women after weight loss. *J. Clin. Endocrinol. Metab.* 2000;85:3338-3342.

[79] Hotamisligil GS. Adipose expression of tumor necrosis factor: direct role in obesity-linked insulin resistance. *Science* 1993:259:87-91.

[80] Kern PA, Saghizadeh M, Ong JM, Bosch RJ, Deem R, Simsolo RB. The expression of tumor necrosis factor in human adipose tissue: regulation by obesity, weight loss, and relationship to lipoprotein lipase. *J. Clin. Invest.* 1995:95:2111-2119.

[81] Otero M, Lego R, Lago F, el al. Leptin, from fat to inflammation: old questions and new insights. *FEBS Lett* 2005;579(2):295-301.

[82] Unger RH. Longevity, lipotoxicity, and leptin: the adipocyte defense against feasting and famine. *Biochimie* 2005;87(1):57-64.

[83] Franks PW, Brage S, Luan J, Ekelund U, Rahman M, Farooqi IS, et al. Leptin predicts a worsening of the features of the metabolic syndrome independently of obesity. *Obes. Res.* 2005;13(8):1476-1484.

[84] Ridker PM, Rifai N, Pfeifer MA, Sacks FM, Moye LA, Goldman S, et al. Inflammation, pravastatin, and the risk of coronary events after myocardial infarction in patients with average cholesterol levels. *Circulation* 1998;98(9)839-844.

[85] Ernst E, Resch KL: Fibrinogen as a cardiovascular risk factor: a meta-analysis and review of the literature. *Ann. Intern. Med.* 18:956–963, 1993

[86] Imperatore G, Riccardi G, Iovine C, Rivellese AA, Vaccaro O: Plasma fibrinogen: a new factor of the metabolic syndrome: a population-based study. *Diabetes Care* 21:649–654, 1998

[87] Schram MT, Stehouver CD. Endothelial dysfunction, cellular adhesion molecules and the metabolic syndrome. *Horm. Metab. Res.* 2005;37(suppl 1):49-55.

[88] Potter van Loon BJ, Kluft C, Radder JK, Blankenstein MA, Meinders AE: The cardiovascular risk factor plasminogen activator inhibitor type 1 is related to insulin resistance. *Metabolism* 42:945–949, 1993

[89] Festa A, D'Agostino R Jr, Mykkanen L, Tracy RP, Zaccaro DJ, Hales CN, Haffner SM: Relative contribution of insulin and its precursors to fibrinogen and PAI-1 in a large population with different states of glucose tolerance: the Insulin Resistance Atherosclerosis Study (IRAS). *Arterioscler. Thromb. Vasc. Biol.* 19:562–568, 1999

[90] Dandona P, Aljada A, Chaudhuri A, Mohanty P, Garg R. Metabolic syndrome: a comprehensive perspective based on interactions between obesity, diabetes, and inflammation. *Circulation* 2005;111(11):1448-1454.

[91] Conlan MG, Folsom AR, Finch A, Davis CE, Sorlie P, Marcucci G, et al. Associations of factor VIII and von Willibrand factor with age, race, sex, and risk factors for atherosclerosis: the atherosclerosis risk in communities (ARIC) study. *Thromb. Haemost.* 1993;70:380-385.

[92] Janand-Delenne B, Chagnaud C, Raccah D, Alessi MC, Juhan-Vague I, Vague P. Visceral fat as a main determinant of plasminogen activator inhibitor 1 level in women. *Int. J. Obes. Relat. Metab. Disord.* 1998;22:312-317.

[93] Sakkinen PA, Wahl P, Cushman M, Lweis MR, Tracy RP. Clustering of procoagulation, inflammation, and fibrinolysis variables with metabolic factors in insulin resistance syndrome. *Am. J. Epidemiol.* 2000;152:897-907.

[94] Juhan-Vague I, Pyke SD, Alessi MC, Jespersen J, Haverkate F, Thompson SG. Fibrinolytic factors and the risk of myocardial infarctionor sudden death in patients with angina pectoris: ECAT study group. European concerted action on thrombosis and disabilities. *Circulation* 1996;94:2057-2063.

[95] Bruno G, Cavallo Perin P, Bargero G, et al. Hyperfibrinogenemia and metabolic syndrome in type 2 diabetes: a population-based study. *Diabetes Metab Res Rev* 2001;17(2): 124-130.

[96] Carr ME. Diabetes mellitus: a hypercoagulable state. *J Diabetes Complications* 2001;15(1):44-54.

[97] American Diabetes Association. Type 2 Diabetes in Children. [Consensus Statement]. *Diabetes Care* 2000;23:381-389.

[98] Weiss R, Dziura J, Burgert TS, et al. Obesity and the metabolic syndrome in children and adolescents. *N Engl J Med* 2004;350(230):2362-2374.

[99] Cook DG, Mendall MA, Whincup PH, Carey IM, Ballam L, Morris JE, Miller GJ, Strachan DP: C-reactive protein concentration in children: relationship to adiposity and other cardiovascular risk factors. *Atherosclerosis* 2000;149:139–150.

[100] Visser M, Bouter LM, McQuillan GM, Wener MH, Harris TB: Low-grade systemic inflammation in overweight children. *Pediatrics* 200;107:E13.

[101] Wu DM, Chu NF, Shen MH, Chang JB: Plasma C-reactive protein levels and their relationship to anthropometric and lipid characteristics among children. *J. Clin. Epidemiol.* 2003;56:94–100.

[102] Vikram NK, Misra A, Dwivedi M, Sharma R, Pandey RM, Luthra K, Chatterjee A, Dhingra V, Jailkhani BL, Talwar KK, Guleria R: Correlations of C-reactive protein levels with anthropometric profile, percentage of body fat and lipids in healthy adolescents and young adults in urban North India. *Atherosclerosis* 2003;168:305–313.

[103] Must A, Jacques PF, Dallal GE, Bajema CJ, Dietz WH: Long-term morbidity and mortality of overweight adolescents: a follow-up of the Harvard Growth Study of 1922 to 1935. *N. Engl. J. Med.* 1992;327:1350–1355.

[104] Gungor N, Thompson T, Sutton-Tyrrell K, Janosky J, Arslanian S. Early signs of cardiovascular disease in youth with obesity and type 2 diabetes. *Diabetes Care* 2005;28:1219-1221.

[105] Sorrentino MJ. Implications of the metabolic syndrome: the new epidemic. *Am. J. Cardiol.* 2005;96(4A):3E-7E.

[106] Pritchett AM, Foreyt JP, Mann DL. Treatment of the metabolic syndrome: the impact of lifestyle modification. *Curr. Atheroscler. Rep.* 2005;7(2):95-102.

[107] Esposito K, Marfella R, Ciotola M, Di Palo C, Giugliano F, Giugliano G, D'Armiento M, D'Andrea F, Giugliano D. Effect of a mediterranean-style diet on endothelial dysfunction and markers of vascular inflammation in the metabolic syndrome: a randomized trial. *JAMA* 2004;292(12):1440.

[108] Riserus U, Basu S, Jovinge S, Fredrikson GN, Arnlov J, Vessby B. Supplementation with conjugated linoleic acid causes isomer-dependent oxidative stress and elevated C-reactive protein: a potential link to fatty acid-induced insulin resistance. *Circulation* 2002;106(15):1925-1929.

[109] Luyckx FH, Lefebvre PJ, Scheen AJ. Non-alcoholic steatohepatitis: association with obesity and insulin resistance, and influence of weight loss. *Diabetes Metab.* 2000;26(2):98-106.

[110] Pitsavos C, Panagiotakos DB, Chrysohoou C, Kavouras S, Stefanadis C. The associations between physical activity, inflammation, and coagulation markers, in people with metabolic syndrome: the ATTICA study. *Eur. J. Cardiovasc. Prev. Rehabil.* 2005;12(2):151-158.

[111] Troseid M, Lappegard KT, Claudi T, Damas JK, Morkrid L, Brendberg R, Mollnes TE. Exercise reduces plasma levels of the chemokines MCP-1 and IL-8 in subjects with the metabolic syndrome. *Eur. Heart. J.* 2004;25(4):349-355.

[112] Bray GA, Champagne CM. Obesity and the Metabolic Syndrome: implications for dietetics practitioners. *J. Am. Diet. Assoc.* 2004;104(1):86-89.

[113] Ishizaka N, Ishizaka Y, Toda E, Hashimoto H, Nagai R, Yamakado M. Association between cigarette smoking, metabolic syndrome, and carotid arteriosclerosis in Japanese individuals. *Atherosclerosis.* 2005;181(2):381-388.

[114] Chu JW, Abbasi F, Lamendola C, McLaughlin T, Reaven GM, Tsao PS. Effect of rosiglitazone treatment on circulating vascular and inflammatory markers in insulin-resistant subjects. *Diab. Vasc. Dis. Res.* 2005;2(1):37-41.

[115] Arner P. The adipocyte in insulin reistance: key molecules and the impact of the thiazolidinediones. *TRENDS in Endocrinol. Metab.* 2003;14(3):137-145.

[116] Iushibashi M, Egashira K, Hiasa K, Inoue S, Ni W, Zhao Q, et al. Antiinflammatory and antiarteriosclerotic effects of pioglitazone. *Hypertension* 2002;40:687-693.

[117] Scandinavian Simvastatin Survival Study Group. Randomised trial of cholesterol lowering in 4444 patients with coronary heart disease: the Scandinavian simvastatin survival study (4S). *Lancet* 1994;344:1383-9.

[118] Kinjo K, Sato H, Sakata Y, et al. Relation of C-reactive protein and one-year survival after acute myocardial infarction with versus without statin therapy. *Am J Cardiol* 2005;96(5):617-621.

[119] Elrod JW, Lefer DJ. The effects of statins on endothelium, inflammation, and cardioprotection. *Drugs News Perspect* 2005;18(4):229-236.

[120] Jialal I, Stein D, Balis D, Grundy SM, Adams-Huet B, Devaraj S: Effects of hydroxymethyl glutaryl coenzyme A reductase inhibitor therapy on high sensitive C-reactive protein levels. *Circulation* 2001;103:1933-1935.

[121] Maki KC. Fibrates for treatment of the metabolic syndrome. *Curr. Atheroscler. Rep.* 2004 J;6(1):45-51.

[122] Dagenais NJ, Jamali F. Protective effects of angiotensin II interruption: evidence for antiinflammatory actions. *Pharmacotherapy* 2005;25(9):1213-1229.

[123] Sierra C, de la Sierra A. Antihypertensive, cardiovascular, and pleiotropic effects of angiotensin-receptor blockers. *Curr. Opin. Nephrol. Hypertens.* 2005;14(5):435-441.

[124] American College of Endocrinology (ACE) Position Statement on the Insulin Resistance Syndrome. *Endocr. Pract.* 2003;9(No. 3):236-252.

[125] van Oostrom AJ, van Wijk J, Cabezas MC. Lipaemia, inflammation and atherosclerosis: novel opportunities in the understanding and treatment of atherosclerosis. *Drugs* 2004;64 Suppl 2:19-41.

[126] Garg R, Tripathy D, Dandona P. Insulin resistance as a proinflammatory state: mechanisms, mediators, and therapeutic interventions. *Curr. Drug. Targets.* 2003;4(6):487-492.

In: Inflammation Research Perspectives
Editor: Giacomo T. Romano, pp. 41-59
ISBN: 978-1-60021-845-3

Chapter III

The Central Nervous System and Inflammation: Microglia

Wolfgang J. Streit, Kelly R. Miller and Kryslaine Lopes
Department of Neuroscience, University of Florida, College of Medicine, Gainesville, FL 32610, USA.

1. Introduction

A network of microglial cells extends throughout the central nervous system (CNS) forming a ubiquitous system of endogenous immunocompetent cells (Graeber & Streit, 1990). This pervasive system ensures that every part of the CNS is under continuous surveillance and that any disturbance in homeostasis, regardless of its location, receives immediate attention for it is the role of microglia to provide a first line of defense in response to any kind of acute perturbation or injury. Inflammation is the tissue response to injury, and microglia represent the principal parenchymal cell type involved in the neuroinflammation that occurs inevitably as a result of acute CNS tissue injury. Often an injury, such as trauma or ischemia, directly causes irreversible tissue necrosis that can produce large amounts of tissue debris. Removal of tissue debris is *the* primary and undisputable function of microglial cells, which provide a quintessential source of endogenous CNS macrophages. This appreciation of microglia as brain macrophages has a long history dating as far back as the beginning of the 20th century (Barron, 1995), and it is probably fair to say that the macrophage identity is one of the few facts that is beyond debate when it comes to microglial cell functions. Other aspects of microglial biology have been more controversial, for example, the question of ontogeny, i.e. whether the cells derive from mesoderm or neuroectoderm, was debated for decades but appears to have been resolved in favor of mesoderm (Streit, 2001).

One issue that has received much discussion in the past and continues to remain controversial is the issue of the functional significance of activated microglia, i.e. Are activated microglia harmful or beneficial? (Schenk & Yednock, 2002; Schwartz, 2003). This issue is of paramount importance within the context of neuroinflammation because in recent years the term *neuroinflammation* has come to be used more or less synonymously with *reactive microgliosis* and/or with *microglial activation*. It is therefore essential to understand and define the features that characterize microglial activation, and summarizing these will be one goal of this chapter. A second goal will be to analyze and retrace the developments that have led to the now prevalent notion that neuroinflammation is a key contributory factor in the pathogenesis of neurodegenerative diseases rather than simply a cellular response to tissue perturbation. We will point out significant caveats in this regard. We will make the point that the diversity in experimental approaches involving both *in vivo* and *in vitro* work have created a rather confusing vision of what exactly constitutes an activated microglial cell and what its function may be. While, in theory, there could be multiple states of microglial activation that span the spectrum from beneficial to harmful, there are currently no methods for identifying different functional microglial "isotypes" *in situ*, yet this would be critical for demonstrating supposedly dangerous, activated cells. Moreover, there is a need for distinguishing between truly activated microglia and ostensibly activated microglia because there is now growing evidence from studies in human brain that some seemingly activated cells may, in fact, be degenerating cells (Streit *et al.*, 2004b; Wierzba-Bobrowicz *et al.*, 2004).

2. What is Microglial Activation?

Although neuroscientists in the early decades of the 20th century, such as Nissl and Spielmeyer, and certainly del Rio-Hortega, were keenly aware that microglia undergo transformation into brain macrophages when CNS tissue is destroyed by injury or disease, research reports dealing with activated (or reactive) microglia were rare until the 1970s. Importantly, the term reactive (activated) microglia was coined and used strictly within the context of *in vivo* neuropathological studies investigating the tissue response to CNS injury. As we shall discuss later, "activated microglia" currently is being used in a much broader sense to include, most notably, *in vitro* scenarios which do not mimic the *in vivo* responses for which the term was intended. Thus, "activated microglia" nowadays can have a very different meaning depending on whether it is used by an *in vitro* or an *in vivo* investigator.

Microglia function not only as phagocytes, but are highly dynamic cells that display exceptional morphological and functional plasticity. In the quiescent brain, microglia are described as "resting", based primarily on their morphological characteristics. Contrary to what this classification may suggest, it has long been the working assumption that resting microglia are in fact busy monitoring their microenvironment in an attempt to maintain homeostasis within the CNS. This assumption was confirmed recently through *in vivo* experiments revealing extremely motile processes and protrusions on resting microglia in the living neocortex of mice (Nimmerjahn *et al.*, 2005). Distributed along their processes and on the cell body are a plethora of surface receptors and ion channels, allowing microglia to detect and respond to myriad signals, such as neurotransmitters, neuropeptides, cytokines, chemokines, ions, growth factors and serum derived components like immunoglobulins, thrombin and complement. Upon insult or injury to the brain, microglia become "activated" undergoing phenotypical changes that include hypertrophy, mitosis, as well as changes in immunophenotype and in cytokine/growth factor production.

2.1. Morphology

In accordance with their highly adaptable nature, microglial morphology varies in correlation with unique functional states. Microglia in the normal, healthy brain are approximately 30-40 μm in diameter, smaller than both astrocytes and oligodendrocytes (Raivich *et al.*, 1999). Resting microglia exhibit a stellate morphology in gray matter, while in the white matter they lie in parallel to nerve fibers. Electron microscopy performed in organotypic hippocampal slice culture reveals microglia with oval or elongated nuclei, dense cytoplasm, dense laminar bodies, homogenous droplets, lysosomes, lipofuscin and a granular endoplasmic reticulum (Skibo *et al.*, 2000). Because of their long, highly branched processes, resting microglia are often referred to as "ramified." Primary branches on resting, ramified microglia may extend more than 50 μm in length, with thin finger-like protrusions extending outward sometimes forming bulbous endings (Nimmerjahn *et al.*, 2005; Stence *et al.*, 2001). Furthermore, both Nimmerjahn *et al.*, (2005) and Stence *et al.*, (2001) provide evidence that microglial processes undergo cycles of formation and withdrawal that occur within minutes, thereby resulting in extensive morphological changes within an hour's time.

Upon insult or injury to the brain, microglia undergo a stereotypical, graduated response commensurate with the severity of brain damage incurred. Prior to becoming fully activated, or in the event of a mild perturbation, microglia may take on a hyper-ramified form (Streit *et al.*, 1999). Fully reactive microglia retract their processes and develop an enlarged cell body. Shortened processes exhibit increased thickness proximally and deramification of distal branches. Additionally, experiments performed using the electron microscope describe reactive microglia as having enlarged nuclei and perikaryon, increased size and number of lysosomes and the appearance of phagosomes (Blinzinger & Hager, 1962). Ultimately, activated microglia responding to injury that does not involve frank neuronal degeneration will decrease in number and return to a resting state (Graeber *et al.*, 1989). When brain damage leads to neuronal degeneration, microglia undergo further transformation from an activated phenotype to that of a phagocyte (Streit & Kreutzberg, 1988). In cases of neuronal cell death, microglia with a macrophage appearance can be detected as early as one to four hours post-injury (Kaur & You, 2000; Skibo *et al.*, 2000). Microglial-derived macrophages take on a rounded, amoeboid shape similar to that of peripheral macrophages . When examined under the electron microscope, phagocytic microglia showed abundant lysosomes and phagosomes as well as copious lipid droplets and lipofuscin material (Kaur & You, 2000; Sobaniec-Lotowska, 2005). Further examination revealed oval or round nuclei with dense heterochromatin accumulated under the nuclear envelope and sparse euchromatin. Finally, microglia-derived macrophages customarily revert to a resting phenotype within a few days to weeks, but active macrophages have been found in white matter tracts up to ten years following middle cerebral artery occlusion (Kosel *et al.*, 1997).

2.2. Proliferation

The mitotic potential of microglia in the adult brain was discovered when autoradiographic studies employing [^{3}H] thymidine incorporation showed that microglia undergo mitosis following brain injury (Friede & Johnstone, 1967; Kreutzberg, 1966; Sjostrand, 1971) Microglial proliferation occurred to a much lesser degree in the absence of an injury, likely reflecting normal cell turnover (Dalton et al., 1968; Lawson et al., 1992; Tonchev et al., 2003). Later experiments confirmed that microglia are the only glial cell type to undergo mitosis after facial nerve axotomy in the rat (Graeber et al., 1988b). However, astrocytic proliferation has been reported in other models (Cao et al., 2003; du Bois et al., 1985; Li et al., 2005; McGinn et al., 2004) Despite the variations in experimental injury models, species and strain differences, as well as methods of detection used to assess glial proliferation, mitosis proves to be a prominent and consistent component of the microglial response to injury.

Microglial proliferation has been studied most exhaustively in the facial nerve axotomy model (Cammermeyer, 1965; Fendrick et al., 2005; Graeber et al., 1988b; Kreutzberg, 1966; Streit & Kreutzberg, 1988). This well established injury paradigm is advantageous in the study of microglial activation primarily because there is no direct trauma to the CNS and the blood brain barrier remains intact, providing an opportunity to study purely endogenous glial responses. An additional advantage is that the injury is well tolerated and highly reproducible from animal to animal. Insights gained from studies employing the facial nerve axotomy and other regenerating nerve models, as well as from acute and chronic neural injury models reveal that microglial proliferation begins as early as 12 hours post-lesion (Ziaja & Janeczko, 1999), peaks at approximately three to four days after insult (Kreutzberg, 1966; Ladeby *et al.*, 2005; Sjostrand, 1971; Streit & Kreutzberg, 1988; Stuesse *et al.*, 2000) and declines thereafter. In contrast to the prevailing mitotic response described above, Tonchev et al. (2003) have shown that there is a differential proliferative response exhibited by microglia after ischemic insult in the macaque monkey. As expected, their study showed that microglial proliferation peaks four days after ischemia in the hippocampus, but surprisingly, mitotic activity in the superior temporal gyrus was delayed until 15 days post-injury. There was no significant increase in microglial proliferation in the parahippocampal region or olfactory bulb. This study highlights the fact that microglial responses are highly specialized and context-specific. Furthermore, there is evidence to show that after microglia have proliferated population control is implemented by apoptosis. In models of facial (Jones *et al.*, 1997), as well as hypoglossal and sciatic nerve injuries (Gehrmann & Banati, 1995), apoptosis of microglia was measured using terminal transferase mediated d-UTP nick end labeling (TUNEL) and in situ end labeling (ISEL) and found to occur beginning four to six days after injury and continuing for up to 21 days.

While the proliferative response of microglia is well-documented and characterized, little is known about mechanisms underlying its regulation. The literature abounds with reports of pharmacological agents and/or endogenous chemicals that stimulate or inhibit microglial proliferation *in vitro*, which is not unexpected given the high sensitivity of microglia to their surrounding milieu. However, these findings are difficult to extrapolate to the *in vivo* situation. Upon careful review of current data, a picture emerges of likely common mechanisms governing microglial mitosis *in vivo*. Specifically, it seems that inducers of microglial proliferation could include interleukin-6 (IL-6) (Streit *et al.*, 2000), the neurotrophin NT-3 (Elkabes *et al.*, 1996) and macrophage colony-stimulating factor (M-CSF) (Kloss *et al.*, 1997). Insights into the molecular mechanisms by which these microglial mitogens exert their effects has been gained in the last few years. *In vitro* experiments have shown that GM-CSF activates Hck tyrosine kinase, which in turn activates the phosphatidylinositol 3-kinase/Akt (PI3K/Akt) pathway (Ito *et al.*, 2005; Suh *et al.*, 2005). Additionally, studies have shown that microglial mitosis induced by GM-CSF administration (Koguchi *et al.*, 2003) and cerebral ischemia (Kato *et al.*, 2003) lead to expression of the cell cycle-associated proteins cyclin D1, E, A and cyclin-dependent kinase inhibitor p21 as well as cyclin D1 and cyclin-dependent kinase-4, respectively. Given the fact that Akt is known to activate cyclins (Mirza *et al.*, 2004) these data collectively provide a highly plausible mechanism for GM-CSF induced microglial mitosis.

The macrophage colony-stimulating factors have received considerable attention for their abilities as microglial mitogens, but IL-6 has also come to be thought of as an inducer of glial proliferation. This is not completely surprising given that IL-6 was previously known as "B cell growth factor" for its stimulation of proliferation in B lymphocytes. Studies strongly suggest that IL-6 released from injured neurons serves as a signal for microglial proliferation and activation in general (Kiefer *et al.*, 1993; Streit *et al.*, 2000; Streit *et al.*, 1998). It was shown that there is an early and robust upregulation of IL-6 mRNA following facial nerve injury that precedes the onset of microglial mitosis (Streit *et al.*, 2000). Concordantly, low levels of IL-6 expression were seen in the red nucleus following rubrospinal tractotomy, as well as in the facial nucleus of neonates post-axotomy, both situations wherein microglial proliferation does not occur. Furthermore, experiments performed on IL-6 deficient mice show significantly delayed microglial responses. Specifically, impairment of microglial proliferation was reported in IL-6 -/- mice following facial nerve axotomy (Galiano *et al.*, 2001; Klein *et al.*, 1997) and in the substantia nigra pars compacta (SNpc) after MPTP lesions (Cardenas & Bolin, 2003). Thus, when examining the beneficial proliferative response of microglia to IL-6, we are again reminded of the highly specialized and context-specific reaction of microglia to a molecule that is known to have multiple effects, both pro- and anti-inflammatory.

2.3. Cytokine/Growth Factor Production

Microglial production of cytokines and growth factors is complex and occurs in a heterogeneous and escalating manner. Certain cytokines known to be constitutively expressed by microglia are thought to act in an autocrine fashion, specifically, transforming growth factor β (TGFβ) (Kiefer *et al.*, 1993; Lehrmann *et al.*, 1998), a pleiotropic growth factor. TGFβ has been shown to exert inhibitory effects on microglial phagocytosis (Stoll *et al.*, 2004) and proliferation (Jones *et al.*, 1998), as well as prevent the induction of microglial genes involved in chemotaxis and cell migration, among others (Paglinawan *et al.*, 2003). The list of cytokines, chemokines and growth factors produced by microglia upon activation is extensive (Hanisch, 2002); however, it is important to note that many cytokines exert both positive and negative effects on the CNS and that it is the degree of microglial activation, or severity of neuronal damage, that determines the ensuing cytokine expression patterns. For example, microglia rapidly upregulate IL-1β, IL-6, TNF-α mRNAs following traumatic spinal cord damage (Bartholdi & Schwab, 1997; Streit *et al.*, 1998; Yang *et al.*, 2005), whereas in the regenerating facial nerve injury paradigm mRNAs of TNF-α and IL-1β, both prototypic proinflammatory cytokines, are only minimally elevated and there is no change in M-CSF mRNA (Raivich *et al.*, 1999; Streit *et al.*, 1998). Interleukin-6, which shows prolonged expression after facial axotomy, is rapidly downregulated after spiking initially in spinal cord injury (Streit *et al.*, 1998). Finally, microglial activation resulting from infection, such as viral meningitis or bacteria-induced encephalitis, leads to production of not only those cytokines listed above, but also interferon-γ (IFN-γ) (Frei *et al.*, 1988; Suzuki *et al.*, 2005). IFN-γ acts to promote upregulation of surface molecules like major histocompatibility complex (MHC) class I and II molecules, complement receptors, Fc receptors and CD14, as well as induce the release of cytokines, complement and nitric oxide (NO) (Hanisch, 2002). In addition, IFN-γ acting synergistically with beta-amyloid (Aβ) peptide has been shown experimentally to induce microglial production of the chemokine monocyte chemotactic protein (MCP-1) (Meda *et al.*, 1996). Microglia are capable of producing many additional cytokines, chemokines and neurotrophins not discussed herein and for additional information the interested reader is referred elsewhere (Hanisch, 2002; van Rossum & Hanisch, 2004).

2.4. Immunophenotype

As with all other aspects of microglial biology, surface molecule expression is highly dynamic and exhibits changes in association with various states of microglial activation. Resting microglia constitutively express type three complement receptors (Graeber *et al.*, 1988a), and Fc and macrophage-specific antigen (Perry *et al.*, 1985), as well as CD4 (Perry & Gordon, 1987) and leukocyte common antigen (Akiyama & McGeer, 1990). However, when microglia become activated, there are changes in surface marker expression that suggest changes in cell function. Within 24 hours of activation, microglia express many molecules important for interactions between lymphocytes and antigen-presenting cells. Specifically, they exhibit an upregulation of CR3 (OX-42) expression (Graeber *et al.*, 1988a) accompanied by an increase in IgG-immunoreactivity, thrombospondin, and intercellular adhesion molecule 1 (Kloss *et al.*, 1999; Moller *et al.*, 1996; Raivich *et al.*, 1999). Peak expression of integrin subunits α5 and α 6 occurs at day four post-injury and the αM-subunit at day 1 and again at days 14-42. Furthermore, within three days of CNS injury, proliferating microglia have been shown to express the stem cell antigen CD34 (Ladeby *et al.*, 2005). Consistent with a role as antigen-presenting cells, reactive microglia show enhanced major histocompatibility complex type I and II (MHC I and II) expression during the first week after injury (Streit *et al.*, 1989a, 1989b). Upregulation of MHC I can be detected in all activated microglia, while MHC II expression is restricted primarily to microglia in degenerating white matter tracts (Streit *et al.*, 1989b; Watanabe *et al.*, 1999). Phagocytic microglia are known to display all of the surface molecules previously discussed, as well as the macrophage surface antigens ED1 and ED3 (Graeber *et al.*, 1990). All in all, there is great heterogeneity in microglial immunophenotypes, which can vary with the type and severity of a lesion, the location within the parenchyma (white *versus* grey matter), and perhaps also with the cells' age, as we shall discuss below.

3. What is Neuroinflammation?

Contrary to the statement that inflammation is a "poorly defined concept" (McGeer & McGeer, 2001) general pathology defines it rather clearly and simply as the reaction of living tissues to all forms of injury (Robbins, 1981). Historically, the term "inflammation" was used primarily in the context of non-CNS injuries, but for about ten years now "neuroinflammation" has become a commonly used phrase (Streit *et al.*, 2004a). Before neuroinflammation came into widespread use, neuroscientists used to talk about "reactive gliosis" to describe the endogenous CNS tissue response to acute injury, and it was recognized thirty years ago that microglia are the prevalent cell type associated with an inflammatory response in the brain (Oehmichen & Huber, 1976). Reactive gliosis specifically refers to the activation of microglia and astrocytes that is triggered immediately and inevitably after CNS injury has occurred. However, CNS injury can occur in many different ways and it can vary dramatically in severity. On one extreme could be a traumatic injury of the brain or the spinal cord where direct physical destruction of the tissue results in hemorrhagic necrosis. This type of lesion is accompanied by an extensive breakdown of the blood brain barrier and infiltration of the CNS parenchyma by blood borne leukocytes, primarily neutrophils (Sroga *et al.*, 2003; Streit *et al.*, 1998). Clearly, in this scenario the term "neuroinflammation" is appropriate because the principal features of general pathology that characterize acute inflammation apply: there are profound vascular changes, as well as a polymorphonuclear leukocytic exudate. Together with the rapid activation of glial cells, these changes represent the response of the living tissue to injury and the critical first step in the wound healing process. On the other end of the spectrum of acute CNS injuries lies a subtle, non-lethal and reversible neuronal injury that triggers glial cell activation but does not involve a breakdown of the blood brain barrier and a concomitant leukocytic exudate. This form of "pure" reactive gliosis occurs after an axotomy of motoneurons which results in chromatolysis, the classic example of reversible neuronal injury (Kreutzberg, 1996). Although reactive gliosis could also be called "neuroinflammation" in line with the general definition of inflammation, i.e. the reaction of living tissue to injury, it is more specific and accurate to talk about reactive gliosis in this situation. Most other types of acute CNS injury, including stroke and neurotoxicant-induced damage, fall in between these two extremes of axotomy and traumatic CNS injury exhibiting patterns of neuroinflammation that are blends between reactive gliosis and leukocytic infiltration.

While acute inflammation comprises the immediate and early response to an injurious event and is basically an adaptive response that paves the way for repair of the damaged site, chronic inflammation results from injurious stimuli that are persistent. In the periphery, both acute and chronic inflammation are characterized by leukocytic exudates consisting primarily of polymorphonuclear cells (neutrophils) in the former and mononuclear cells (macrophages, lymphocytes, plasma cells) in the latter. However, in the CNS, due largely to the presence of the blood brain barrier, leukocytic exudates may not be part of chronic neuroinflammation, certainly not in the way the term is currently being used in the context of neurodegenerative diseases (see below). Chronic neuroinflammation is indeed more relevant in the context of CNS disease rather than CNS injury, since "disease" implicitly carries the notion of chronicity. The classic example of chronic neuroinflammation is the autoimmune neuroinflammation that occurs in multiple sclerosis. Although the underlying cause(s) of MS have not been elucidated, it is probably safe to say that the persistent injurious stimulus that accounts for MS neuroinflammation is a myelin-related protein that has escaped self-tolerance and become an autoantigen. Consistent with the chronic persistence of this CNS autoantigen is a persistent accumulation of blood-derived mononuclear leukocytes in the CNS parenchyma, which mirrors the presence of leukocytic exudates in peripheral autoimmune diseases, such as rheumatoid arthritis or polymyositis.

Most infectious diseases of the CNS, if they are not cleared, produce chronic neuroinflammation. The most important example in modern times is infection with the human immunodeficiency virus (HIV) which is known to enter and remain in the CNS *via* myelomonocytic cells, such as monocytes, perivascular cells, and microglia (Garden, 2002). However, HIV infection is uniquely different from most other infectious diseases affecting the CNS in that the virus targets and disables precisely those cells that are key players in neuroinflammation – microglia and T lymphocytes. It therefore comes as no surprise that prominent T cell infiltrates do not occur in HIV encephalopathy. Similarly, prion diseases, which represent another infectious CNS disease of major current interest, are atypical with regard to neuroinflammation (Eikelenboom *et al.*, 2002; Perry *et al.*, 2002). Microglial activation appears to be the most prominent component of the neuroinflammation associated with prion diseases, although there are a few reports describing T cell infiltration as well (Betmouni *et al.*, 1996; Lewicki *et al.*, 2003).

As an interesting parallel to HIV infection, prions seem to infect microglial cells in addition to neurons and this may help explain the unusual patterns of neuroinflammation that becomes manifest not only in atypical cellular infiltrates but also in unusual cytokine profiles (Baker & Manuelidis, 2003). Thus, both HIV and prion infections probably produce an altered microglial physiology that is likely to translate into microglial dysfunction, which could be a contributing factor in the development of dementia that occurs in these conditions.

3.1. Reactive Microgliosis versus Chronic Neuroinflammation in Neurodegenerative Diseases

Neurodegenerative diseases, particularly Alzheimer's disease (AD) and amyotrophic lateral sclerosis (ALS), but also Parkinson's and Huntington's disease lack the prominent infiltrates of blood-derived mononuclear cells that characterize autoimmune diseases and can therefore not be categorized as chronic inflammatory conditions. On the other hand, there is abundant evidence to show that many substances involved in the promotion of inflammatory processes can be detected in the CNS of patients with neurodegenerative diseases, and some of these proinflammatory mediators appear to be increased relative to non-diseased controls. By far the bulk of this body of evidence is related to studies in AD (Akiyama *et al.*, 2000), and we therefore discuss the issue of reactive microgliosis *versus* chronic neuroinflammation within the context of AD. What distinguishes AD from other neurodegenerative diseases is the widespread presence of extracellular deposits of amyloid in senile plaques. Senile plaques are present in the AD brain in different stages of maturity ranging from diffuse to dense core or neuritic, but they all contain the amyloid beta protein (Aβ). Aβ is a pathological protein that tends to form aggregates creating insoluble extracellular deposits which attract microglial cells, as suggested by the clustering of microglia at sites of Aβ deposition (Streit, 2004). There is compelling evidence from experimental studies in animals to support the idea that microglia phagocytose and attempt to degrade amyloid (Frautschy *et al.*, 1992; Weldon *et al.*, 1998), but whether they do so effectively in humans with AD is questionable. In fact, a very recent report strongly suggests that they do not (Fiala *et al.*, 2005). A key question within the current context is, Does the presence of amyloid in AD brain represent a persistent injurious stimulus that incites chronic neuroinflammation? Differently put, Does phagocytosis or attempted phagocytosis of amyloid by microglia constitute chronic neuroinflammation? The answer to this is not obvious, because it is not certain whether amyloid represents an injurious stimulus or a consequence of an injury. Direct injection of amyloid into the brain does not produce neurodegeneration or overt neuronal injury (Weldon *et al.*, 1998), and transgenic mice that overexpress the amyloid precursor protein and develop amyloid deposits do not show neurodegenerative changes, such as neurofibrillary tangles (Irizarry *et al.*, 1997). At the same time, there is evidence that shows increased presence of Aβ and amyloid precursor protein after traumatic head injury (Smith *et al.*, 2003) suggesting that Aβ production is enhanced as a result of CNS injury. It is therefore conceivable that the increased presence of Aβ in the AD brain is a result of ongoing neuronal damage rather than the cause of it, but a final answer as to whether Aβ is pathogenic or merely a byproduct of the disease process must await further studies. What seems to be indisputable at this point in time is that amyloid, when deposited extracellularly, induces a reactive glial response by both astrocytes and microglia (Frautschy *et al.*, 1998; Irizarry *et al.*, 1997). For the time being it may therefore be most accurate and objective to speak of reactive gliosis rather than of chronic inflammation when considering the innate glial response to amyloid. This view is entirely compatible with the large body of evidence that shows enhanced presence of a wide array of proinflammatory substances in the AD brain because anytime reactive gliosis occurs, cytokines and other proinflammatory substances are produced as part of the mobilization of the endogenous defense system (Raivich *et al.*, 1999; Streit *et al.*, 2000; Streit *et al.*, 1998). In conclusion, while it is reasonable and acceptable to include reactive microgliosis under the more general heading of neuroinflammation since reactive microglia are cells responding to CNS injury, it is inappropriate at this point to classify neurodegenerative diseases, particularly AD, as chronic inflammatory conditions because these disorders do not show leukocytic exudates. Moreover, there is no compelling evidence to show that the reactive gliosis that occurs in AD or other neurodegenerative diseases is causing any loss of neurons or synapses that accounts for cognitive deficits and dementia. Nonetheless, it appears that a large number of researchers has embraced the idea that microgliosis in AD is indeed contributing to neurodegeneration. In the following, we attempt to retrace the evolution of this neuroinflammation theory of AD pathogenesis hoping that in the process we are able to shed some new light on the relationship between microglia and CNS inflammation.

3.2. Evolution of the Neuroinflammation Hypothesis

In the early 1980s amidst newfound excitement over astrocytes and oligodendrocytes which stemmed in part from the availability of new methods for maintaining these glial cells *in vitro* (McCarthy & de Vellis, 1980), microglia had become the forgotten third element of Cajal. However, it wasn't long before methods were published that described methods for culturing microglia (Giulian & Baker, 1986). At about the same time, advances were also being made on a different front, namely, the *in vivo* visualization of microglia using immunohistochemical and lectin histochemical procedures (Mannoji *et al.*, 1986; Perry *et al.*, 1985; Streit & Kreutzberg, 1987). Together, the simultaneous developments of both *in vitro* and *in vivo* methodologies for studying microglia gave rise to an upsurge in the numbers of papers published on microglia (Graeber, 1994), a trend that has continued to the present day . However, the take-home messages that emerged from the two different lines of investigations were quite divergent. While investigators working *in vivo* produced primarily descriptive data that provided details on morphological and phenotypic changes occurring on activated microglia as they were responding *in situ* to a variety of experimental CNS lesions, others who worked primarily *in vitro* were quick to report findings with perceived functional significance for the activity of microglia *in vivo*, namely, that activated microglia function as potentially harmful immune effector cells (Boje & Arora, 1992; Giulian, 1987). We can now state with confidence that this was a fallacy, not only because other cell culture studies have reported neurotrophic effects of *in vitro* activated microglia (Elkabes *et al.*, 1996; Nagata *et al.*, 1993), but primarily because the methods that were and are still being used for inducing microglial activation *in vitro* do not simulate *in vivo* conditions where neuronal injury or death is a trigger for microglial activation. Bacterial endotoxin (LPS) was and is the most commonly employed microglial stimulant to generate so-called activated microglia *in vitro*, but the LPS stimulation paradigm at best simulates a fulminant bacterial infection of the brain parenchyma, which is uncommon clinically and usually occurs only in severely immunocompromised patients. Moreover, those unstimulated microglial cells *in vitro* that are subjected to LPS treatment are already activated as they have already undergone transformation into macrophages following dissociation and trituration of brain tissue which is a necessary first step in the preparation of primary microglial cell cultures. Thus, unstimulated microglia *in vitro* are not at all like resting microglia *in* vivo; they are much more similar to microglia-derived macrophages that accumulate after extensive brain damage. The stimulation of these cells with LPS or other immunostimulatory agents *in vitro* essentially produces superactivated cells that have no known counterpart *in vivo*. Notwithstanding these serious shortcomings, cell culture studies gained widespread acceptance and were crucial in promoting a perception of microglia as harmful, neurotoxin-producing immune effector cells (Giulian *et al.*, 1993). Many cell culture studies have also used amyloid as a microglial activator and although there is little doubt that amyloid exposure does indeed alter microglial functional states *in vitro* (Araujo & Cotman, 1992; Korotzer *et al.*, 1993; McDonald *et al.*, 1997; Meda *et al.*, 1995), a causal link between amyloid-activated microglia and the development of neurofibrillary degeneration has not been established. In fact, the aforementioned *in vivo* studies using APP overexpressing mice

(Irizarry *et al.*, 1997) that fail to develop neurofibrillary degeneration provide a very strong argument against such a connection.

Another issue that contributed significantly to the neuroinflammation hypothesis concerns the somewhat arbitrary identification of activated microglia in human brain. Investigators performing post-mortem histopathological studies in the late 1980s were quick to identify microglia as activated based on the fact that the cells were positive for MHC antigens (McGeer *et al.*, 1987; Rogers *et al.*, 1988). Although this seemed to be in concordance with experimental animal studies where reactive microgliosis was usually accompanied by an increase in MHC antigen expression, we know now that MHC expression alone is not a good method for identifying activated microglia. In human brain, MHC antigen expression is seen frequently on microglia exhibiting a resting (ramified) non-activated morphology (Streit *et al.*, 2004b). In addition, MHC expression is virtually absent from microglia in very young humans (Streit & Sparks, 1997), as well as from young rodents and acute injury in neonatal rats produces very limited expression of these microglial markers on activated cells (Morioka & Streit, 1991). On the other hand, MHC expression clearly increases with normal, non-pathological aging on microglia in all species examined thus far, including humans (Perry *et al.*, 1993; Rogers *et al.*, 1988; Sheffield & Berman, 1998; Streit & Sparks, 1997). In light of these observations, it seems much more likely that MHC expression is a marker of cell maturation rather than of cell activation.

Another factor that contributed significantly to the propagation of the neuroinflammation hypothesis is found in epidemiological data from arthritis patients taking anti-inflammatory drugs who seemed to have a lower incidence of AD, which in turn has led to the suggestion that anti-inflammatory drugs could be used in the treatment and/or prevention of AD (McGeer *et al.*, 1996). Since then clinical trials have been conducted with NSAIDs, but thus far no benefits of these drugs for AD prevention have been reported (Aisen *et al.*, 2003). A significant caveat in the epidemiological studies analyzed by McGeer et al. (1996) is that the studies reviewed were largely focused on rheumatoid arthritis, which is a truly inflammatory and autoimmune condition that has its usual onset in young adults (Robbins, 1981). This condition is to be distinguished from osteoarthritis, which is aging-related, degenerative joint disease characterized by minimal inflammation. Osteoarthritis seems like a condition that is much more analogous to AD than rheumatoid arthritis (which might be likened to multiple sclerosis), and it would therefore appear to be more relevant to ask if any treatments for osteoarthritris might be beneficial for AD.

4. Summary

In closing, the idea that neuroinflammation contributes to neurodegeneration in conditions other than autoimmune diseases was borne out of misconceptions about the nature and function of activated microglia. We are inclined to maintain the original perception of activated microglia as cells that are reacting to a disturbance of tissue homeostasis. Accordingly, use of the term should be limited to *in situ* investigations of tissues where the identification of activated microglia can be performed reliably using a combination of morphologic and immunophenotypic criteria.

References

Aisen, P. S., Schafer, K. A., Grundman, M., Pfeiffer, E., Sano, M., Davis, K. L., Farlow, M. R., Jin, S., Thomas, R. G. & Thal, L. J. (2003). Effects of rofecoxib or naproxen vs placebo on Alzheimer disease progression: a randomized controlled trial. *Jama*, 289(21), 2819-2826.

Akiyama, H., Barger, S., Barnum, S., Bradt, B., Bauer, J., Cole, G. M., Cooper, N. R., Eikelenboom, P., Emmerling, M., Fiebich, B. L., Finch, C. E., Frautschy, S., Griffin, W. S., Hampel, H., Hull, M., Landreth, G., Lue, L., Mrak, R., Mackenzie, I. R., McGeer, P. L., O'Banion, M. K., Pachter, J., Pasinetti, G., Plata-Salaman, C., Rogers, J., Rydel, R., Shen, Y., Streit, W., Strohmeyer, R., Tooyoma, I., Van Muiswinkel, F. L., Veerhuis, R., Walker, D., Webster, S., Wegrzyniak, B., Wenk, G. & Wyss-Coray, T. (2000). Inflammation and Alzheimer's disease. *Neurobiol Aging*, 21(3), 383-421.

Akiyama, H. & McGeer, P. L. (1990). Brain microglia constitutively express beta-2 integrins. *J Neuroimmunol*, 30(1), 81-93.

Araujo, D. M. & Cotman, C. W. (1992). Beta-amyloid stimulates glial cells in vitro to produce growth factors that accumulate in senile plaques in Alzheimer's disease. *Brain Res*, 569(1), 141-145.

Baker, C. A. & Manuelidis, L. (2003). Unique inflammatory RNA profiles of microglia in Creutzfeldt-Jakob disease. *Proc Natl Acad Sci U S A*, 100(2), 675-679.

Barron, K. D. (1995). The microglial cell. A historical review. *J Neurol Sci*, 134 Suppl, 57-68.

Bartholdi, D. & Schwab, M. E. (1997). Expression of pro-inflammatory cytokine and chemokine mRNA upon experimental spinal cord injury in mouse: an in situ hybridization study. *Eur J Neurosci*, 9(7), 1422-1438.

Betmouni, S., Perry, V. H. & Gordon, J. L. (1996). Evidence for an early inflammatory response in the central nervous system of mice with scrapie. *Neuroscience*, 74(1), 1-5.

Blinzinger, K. & Hager, H. (1962). [Electron microscope studies on the fine structure of resting and progressive microglia cells in the mammalian brain.]. *Beitr Pathol Anat*, 127, 173-192.

Boje, K. M. & Arora, P. K. (1992). Microglial-produced nitric oxide and reactive nitrogen oxides mediate neuronal cell death. *Brain Res*, 587(2), 250-256.

Cammermeyer, J. (1965). Juxtavascular karyokinesis and microglia cell proliferation during retrograde reaction in the mouse facial nucleus. *Ergeb Anat Entwicklungsgesch*, 38, 1-22.

Cao, Y., Gunn, A. J., Bennet, L., Wu, D., George, S., Gluckman, P. D., Shao, X. M. & Guan, J. (2003). Insulin-like growth factor (IGF)-1 suppresses oligodendrocyte caspase-3 activation and increases glial proliferation after ischemia in near-term fetal sheep. *J Cereb Blood Flow Metab*, 23(6), 739-747.

Cardenas, H. & Bolin, L. M. (2003). Compromised reactive microgliosis in MPTP-lesioned IL-6 KO mice. *Brain Res*, 985(1), 89-97.

Dalton, M. M., Hommes, O. R. & Leblond, C. P. (1968). Correlation of glial proliferation with age in the mouse brain. *J Comp Neurol*, 134(4), 397-400.

du Bois, M., Bowman, P. D. & Goldstein, G. W. (1985). Cell proliferation after ischemic injury in gerbil brain. An immunocytochemical and autoradiographic study. *Cell Tissue Res*, 242(1), 17-23.

Eikelenboom, P., Bate, C., Van Gool, W. A., Hoozemans, J. J., Rozemuller, J. M., Veerhuis, R. & Williams, A. (2002). Neuroinflammation in Alzheimer's disease and prion disease. *Glia*, 40(2), 232-239.

Elkabes, S., DiCicco-Bloom, E. M. & Black, I. B. (1996). Brain microglia/macrophages express neurotrophins that selectively regulate microglial proliferation and function. *J Neurosci*, 16(8), 2508-2521.

Fendrick, S. E., Miller, K. R. & Streit, W. J. (2005). Minocycline does not inhibit microglia proliferation or neuronal regeneration in the facial nucleus following crush injury. *Neurosci Lett*, 385(3), 220-223.

Fiala, M., Lin, J., Ringman, J., Kermani-Arab, V., Tsao, G., Patel, A., Lossinsky, A. S., Graves, M. C., Gustavson, A., Sayre, J., Sofroni, E., Suarez, T., Chiappelli, F. & Bernard, G. (2005). Ineffective phagocytosis of amyloid-beta by macrophages of Alzheimer's disease patients. *J Alzheimers Dis*, 7(3), 221-232.

Frautschy, S. A., Cole, G. M. & Baird, A. (1992). Phagocytosis and deposition of vascular beta-amyloid in rat brains injected with Alzheimer beta-amyloid. *Am J Pathol*, 140(6), 1389-1399.

Frautschy, S. A., Yang, F., Irrizarry, M., Hyman, B., Saido, T. C., Hsiao, K. & Cole, G. M. (1998). Microglial response to amyloid plaques in APPsw transgenic mice. *Am J Pathol*, 152(1), 307-317.

Frei, K., Leist, T. P., Meager, A., Gallo, P., Leppert, D., Zinkernagel, R. M. & Fontana, A. (1988). Production of B cell stimulatory factor-2 and interferon gamma in the central nervous system during viral meningitis and encephalitis. Evaluation in a murine model infection and in patients. *J Exp Med*, 168(1), 449-453.

Friede, R. L. & Johnstone, M. A. (1967). Responses of thymidine labeling of nuclei in gray matter and nerve following sciatic transection. *Acta Neuropathol* (Berl), 7(3), 218-231.

Galiano, M., Liu, Z. Q., Kalla, R., Bohatschek, M., Koppius, A., Gschwendtner, A., Xu, S., Werner, A., Kloss, C. U., Jones, L. L., Bluethmann, H. & Raivich, G. (2001). Interleukin-6 (IL6) and cellular response to facial nerve injury: effects on lymphocyte recruitment, early microglial activation and axonal outgrowth in IL6-deficient mice. *Eur J Neurosci*, 14(2), 327-341.

Garden, G. A. (2002). Microglia in human immunodeficiency virus-associated neurodegeneration. *Glia*, 40(2), 240-251.

Gehrmann, J. & Banati, R. B. (1995). Microglial turnover in the injured CNS: activated microglia undergo delayed DNA fragmentation following peripheral nerve injury. *J Neuropathol Exp Neurol*, 54(5), 680-688.

Giulian, D. (1987). Ameboid microglia as effectors of inflammation in the central nervous system. *J Neurosci Res*, 18(1), 155 171, 132-153.

Giulian, D. & Baker, T. J. (1986). Characterization of ameboid microglia isolated from developing mammalian brain. *J Neurosci*, 6(8), 2163-2178.

Giulian, D., Corpuz, M., Chapman, S., Mansouri, M. & Robertson, C. (1993). Reactive mononuclear phagocytes release neurotoxins after ischemic and traumatic injury to the central nervous system. *J Neurosci Res*, 36(6), 681-693.

Graeber, M. B. (1994). Development of the microglia literature. *Neuropathol Appl Neurobiol*, 20(2), 215-216.

Graeber, M. B. & Streit, W. J. (1990). Microglia: immune network in the CNS. *Brain Pathol*, 1(1), 2-5.

Graeber, M. B., Streit, W. J., Kiefer, R., Schoen, S. W. & Kreutzberg, G. W. (1990). New expression of myelomonocytic antigens by microglia and perivascular cells following lethal motor neuron injury. *J Neuroimmunol*, 27(2-3), 121-132.

Graeber, M. B., Streit, W. J. & Kreutzberg, G. W. (1988a). Axotomy of the rat facial nerve leads to increased CR3 complement receptor expression by activated microglial cells. *J Neurosci Res*, 21(1), 18-24.

Graeber, M. B., Streit, W. J. & Kreutzberg, G. W. (1989). Formation of microglia-derived brain macrophages is blocked by adriamycin. *Acta Neuropathol* (Berl), 78(4), 348-358.

Graeber, M. B., Tetzlaff, W., Streit, W. J. & Kreutzberg, G. W. (1988b). Microglial cells but not astrocytes undergo mitosis following rat facial nerve axotomy. *Neurosci Lett*, 85(3), 317-321.

Hanisch, U. K. (2002). Microglia as a source and target of cytokines. *Glia*, 40(2), 140-155.

Irizarry, M. C., McNamara, M., Fedorchak, K., Hsiao, K. & Hyman, B. T. (1997). APPSw transgenic mice develop age-related A beta deposits and neuropil abnormalities, but no neuronal loss in CA1. *J Neuropathol Exp Neurol*, 56(9), 965-973.

Ito, S., Sawada, M., Haneda, M., Fujii, S., Oh-Hashi, K., Kiuchi, K., Takahashi, M. & Isobe, K. (2005). Amyloid-beta peptides induce cell proliferation and macrophage colony-stimulating factor expression via the PI3-kinase/Akt pathway in cultured Ra2 microglial cells. *FEBS Lett*, 579(9), 1995-2000.

Jones, L. L., Banati, R. B., Graeber, M. B., Bonfanti, L., Raivich, G. & Kreutzberg, G. W. (1997). Population control of microglia: does apoptosis play a role? *J Neurocytol*, 26(11), 755-770.

Jones, L. L., Kreutzberg, G. W. & Raivich, G. (1998). Transforming growth factor beta's 1, 2 and 3 inhibit proliferation of ramified microglia on an astrocyte monolayer. *Brain Research*, 795(1-2), 301-306.

Kato, H., Takahashi, A. & Itoyama, Y. (2003). Cell cycle protein expression in proliferating microglia and astrocytes following transient global cerebral ischemia in the rat. *Brain Res Bull*, 60(3), 215-221.

Kaur, C. & You, Y. (2000). Ultrastructure and function of the amoeboid microglial cells in the periventricular white matter in postnatal rat brain following a hypoxic exposure. *Neurosci Lett*, 290(1), 17-20.

Kiefer, R., Lindholm, D. & Kreutzberg, G. W. (1993). Interleukin-6 and transforming growth factor-beta 1 mRNAs are induced in rat facial nucleus following motoneuron axotomy. *Eur J Neurosci*, 5(7), 775-781.

Klein, M. A., Moller, J. C., Jones, L. L., Bluethmann, H., Kreutzberg, G. W. & Raivich, G. (1997). Impaired neuroglial activation in interleukin-6 deficient mice. *Glia*, 19(3), 227-233.

Kloss, C. U., Kreutzberg, G. W. & Raivich, G. (1997). Proliferation of ramified microglia on an astrocyte monolayer: characterization of stimulatory and inhibitory cytokines. *J Neurosci Res*, 49(2), 248-254.

Kloss, C. U., Werner, A., Klein, M. A., Shen, J., Menuz, K., Probst, J. C., Kreutzberg, G. W. & Raivich, G. (1999). Integrin family of cell adhesion molecules in the injured brain: regulation and cellular localization in the normal and regenerating mouse facial motor nucleus. *J Comp Neurol*, 411(1), 162-178.

Koguchi, K., Nakatsuji, Y., Okuno, T., Sawada, M. & Sakoda, S. (2003). Microglial cell cycle-associated proteins control microglial proliferation in vivo and in vitro and are regulated by GM-CSF and density-dependent inhibition. *J Neurosci Res*, 74(6), 898-905.

Korotzer, A. R., Pike, C. J. & Cotman, C. W. (1993). beta-Amyloid peptides induce degeneration of cultured rat microglia. *Brain Res*, 624(1-2), 121-125.

Kosel, S., Egensperger, R., Bise, K., Arbogast, S., Mehraein, P. & Graeber, M. B. (1997). Long-lasting perivascular accumulation of major histocompatibility complex class II-positive lipophages in the spinal cord of stroke patients: possible relevance for the immune privilege of the brain. *Acta Neuropathol* (Berl), 94(6), 532-538.

Kreutzberg, G. W. (1966). Autoradiographische Untersuchung uber die Beteiligung von Gliazellen an der axonalen Reaktion im Facialiskern der Ratte. *Acta Neuropathol* (Berl), 7, 149-161.

Kreutzberg, G. W. (1996). Microglia: a sensor for pathological events in the CNS. *Trends Neurosci*, 19(8), 312-318.

Ladeby, R., Wirenfeldt, M., Dalmau, I., Gregersen, R., Garcia-Ovejero, D., Babcock, A., Owens, T. & Finsen, B. (2005). Proliferating resident microglia express the stem cell antigen CD34 in response to acute neural injury. *Glia*, 50(2), 121-131.

Lawson, L. J., Perry, V. H. & Gordon, S. (1992). Turnover of resident microglia in the normal adult mouse brain. *Neuroscience*, 48(2), 405-415.

Lehrmann, E., Kiefer, R., Christensen, T., Toyka, K. V., Zimmer, J., Diemer, N. H., Hartung, H. P. & Finsen, B. (1998). Microglia and macrophages are major sources of locally produced transforming growth factor-beta1 after transient middle cerebral artery occlusion in rats. *Glia*, 24(4), 437-448.

Lewicki, H., Tishon, A., Homann, D., Mazarguil, H., Laval, F., Asensio, V. C., Campbell, I. L., DeArmond, S., Coon, B., Teng, C., Gairin, J. E. & Oldstone, M. B. (2003). T cells infiltrate the brain in murine and human transmissible spongiform encephalopathies. *J Virol*, 77(6), 3799-3808.

Li, Y., Chen, J., Zhang, C. L., Wang, L., Lu, D., Katakowski, M., Gao, Q., Shen, L. H., Zhang, J., Lu, M. & Chopp, M. (2005). Gliosis and brain remodeling after treatment of stroke in rats with marrow stromal cells. *Glia*, 49(3), 407-417.

Mannoji, H., Yeger, H. & Becker, L. E. (1986). A specific histochemical marker (lectin Ricinus communis agglutinin-1) for normal human microglia, and application to routine histopathology. *Acta Neuropathol* (Berl), 71(3-4), 341-343.

McCarthy, K. D. & de Vellis, J. (1980). Preparation of separate astroglial and oligodendroglial cell cultures from rat cerebral tissue. *J Cell Biol*, 85(3), 890-902.

McDonald, D. R., Brunden, K. R. & Landreth, G. E. (1997). Amyloid fibrils activate tyrosine kinase-dependent signaling and superoxide production in microglia. *J Neurosci*, 17(7), 2284-2294.

McGeer, P. L., Itagaki, S., Tago, H. & McGeer, E. G. (1987). Reactive microglia in patients with senile dementia of the Alzheimer type are positive for the histocompatibility glycoprotein HLA-DR. *Neurosci Lett*, 79(1-2), 195-200.

McGeer, P. L. & McGeer, E. G. (2001). Inflammation, autotoxicity and Alzheimer disease. *Neurobiol Aging*, 22(6), 799-809.

McGeer, P. L., Schulzer, M. & McGeer, E. G. (1996). Arthritis and anti-inflammatory agents as possible protective factors for Alzheimer's disease: a review of 17 epidemiologic studies. *Neurology*, 47(2), 425-432.

McGinn, M. J., Sun, D., Schneider, S. L., Alexander, J. K. & Colello, R. J. (2004). Epidermal growth factor-induced cell proliferation in the adult rat striatum. *Brain Res*, 1007(1-2), 29-38.

Meda, L., Bernasconi, S., Bonaiuto, C., Sozzani, S., Zhou, D., Otvos, L., Jr., Mantovani, A., Rossi, F. & Cassatella, M. A. (1996). Beta-amyloid (25-35) peptide and IFN-gamma synergistically induce the production of the chemotactic cytokine MCP-1/JE in monocytes and microglial cells. *J Immunol*, 157(3), 1213-1218.

Meda, L., Cassatella, M. A., Szendrei, G. I., Otvos, L., Jr., Baron, P., Villalba, M., Ferrari, D. & Rossi, F. (1995). Activation of microglial cells by beta-amyloid protein and interferon-gamma. *Nature*, 374(6523), 647-650.

Mirza, A. M., Gysin, S., Malek, N., Nakayama, K., Roberts, J. M. & McMahon, M. (2004). Cooperative regulation of the cell division cycle by the protein kinases RAF and AKT. *Mol Cell Biol*, 24(24), 10868-10881.

Moller, J. C., Klein, M. A., Haas, S., Jones, L. L., Kreutzberg, G. W. & Raivich, G. (1996). Regulation of thrombospondin in the regenerating mouse facial motor nucleus. *Glia*, 17(2), 121-132.

Morioka, T. & Streit, W. J. (1991). Expression of immunomolecules on microglial cells following neonatal sciatic nerve axotomy. *J Neuroimmunol*, 35(1-3), 21-30.

Nagata, K., Takei, N., Nakajima, K., Saito, H. & Kohsaka, S. (1993). Microglial conditioned medium promotes survival and development of cultured mesencephalic neurons from embryonic rat brain. *J Neurosci Res*, 34(3), 357-363.

Nimmerjahn, A., Kirchhoff, F. & Helmchen, F. (2005). Resting microglial cells are highly dynamic surveillants of brain parenchyma in vivo. *Science*, 308(5726), 1314-1318.

Oehmichen, M. & Huber, H. (1976). Reactive microglia with membrane features of mononuclear phagocytes. *J Neuropathol Exp Neurol*, 35(1), 30-39.

Paglinawan, R., Malipiero, U., Schlapbach, R., Frei, K., Reith, W. & Fontana, A. (2003). TGFbeta directs gene expression of activated microglia to an anti-inflammatory phenotype strongly focusing on chemokine genes and cell migratory genes. *Glia*, 44(3), 219-231.

Perry, V. H., Cunningham, C. & Boche, D. (2002). Atypical inflammation in the central nervous system in prion disease. *Curr Opin Neurol*, 15(3), 349-354.

Perry, V. H. & Gordon, S. (1987). Modulation of CD4 antigen on macrophages and microglia in rat brain. *J Exp Med*, 166(4), 1138-1143.

Perry, V. H., Hume, D. A. & Gordon, S. (1985). Immunohistochemical localization of macrophages and microglia in the adult and developing mouse brain. *Neuroscience*, 15(2), 313-326.

Perry, V. H., Matyszak, M. K. & Fearn, S. (1993). Altered antigen expression of microglia in the aged rodent CNS. *Glia*, 7(1), 60-67.

Raivich, G., Bohatschek, M., Kloss, C. U., Werner, A., Jones, L. L. & Kreutzberg, G. W. (1999). Neuroglial activation repertoire in the injured brain: graded response, molecular mechanisms and cues to physiological function. *Brain Res Brain Res Rev*, 30(1), 77-105.

Robbins, S. L., Angell, M., Kumar, V. (1981). *Basic Pathology* (3rd ed.). Philadelphia: W.B. Saunders.

Rogers, J., Luber-Narod, J., Styren, S. D. & Civin, W. H. (1988). Expression of immune system-associated antigens by cells of the human central nervous system: relationship to the pathology of Alzheimer's disease. *Neurobiol Aging*, 9(4), 339-349.

Schenk, D. B. & Yednock, T. (2002). The role of microglia in Alzheimer's disease: friend or foe? *Neurobiol Aging*, 23(5), 677-679; discussion 683-674.

Schwartz, M. (2003). Macrophages and microglia in central nervous system injury: are they helpful or harmful? *J Cereb Blood Flow Metab*, 23(4), 385-394.

Sheffield, L. G. & Berman, N. E. (1998). Microglial expression of MHC class II increases in normal aging of nonhuman primates. *Neurobiol Aging*, 19(1), 47-55.

Sjostrand, J. (1971). Neuroglial proliferation in the hypoglossal nucleus after nerve injury. *Exp Neurol*, 30(1), 178-189.

Skibo, G. G., Nikonenko, I. R., Savchenko, V. L. & McKanna, J. A. (2000). Microglia in organotypic hippocampal slice culture and effects of hypoxia: ultrastructure and lipocortin-1 immunoreactivity. *Neuroscience*, 96(2), 427-438.

Smith, D. H., Uryu, K., Saatman, K. E., Trojanowski, J. Q. & McIntosh, T. K. (2003). Protein accumulation in traumatic brain injury. *Neuromolecular Med*, 4(1-2), 59-72.

Sobaniec-Lotowska, M. E. (2005). A transmission electron microscopic study of microglia/macrophages in the hippocampal cortex and neocortex following chronic exposure to valproate. *Int J Exp Pathol*, 86(2), 91-96.

Sroga, J. M., Jones, T. B., Kigerl, K. A., McGaughy, V. M. & Popovich, P. G. (2003). Rats and mice exhibit distinct inflammatory reactions after spinal cord injury. *J Comp Neurol*, 462(2), 223-240.

Stence, N., Waite, M. & Dailey, M. E. (2001). Dynamics of microglial activation: a confocal time-lapse analysis in hippocampal slices. *Glia* (33), 256-266.

Stoll, G., Schroeter, M., Jander, S., Siebert, H., Wollrath, A., Kleinschnitz, C. & Bruck, W. (2004). Lesion-associated expression of transforming growth factor-beta-2 in the rat nervous system: evidence for down-regulating the phagocytic activity of microglia and macrophages. *Brain Pathol*, 14(1), 51-58.

Streit, W. J. (2001). Microglia and macrophages in the developing CNS. *Neurotoxicology*, 22(5), 619-624.

Streit, W. J. (2004). Microglia and Alzheimer's disease pathogenesis. *J Neurosci Res*, 77(1), 1-8.

Streit, W. J., Graeber, M. B. & Kreutzberg, G. W. (1989a). Expression of Ia antigen on perivascular and microglial cells after sublethal and lethal motor neuron injury. *Exp Neurol*, 105(2), 115-126.

Streit, W. J., Graeber, M. B. & Kreutzberg, G. W. (1989b). Peripheral nerve lesion produces increased levels of major histocompatibility complex antigens in the central nervous system. *J Neuroimmunol*, 21(2-3), 117-123.

Streit, W. J., Hurley, S. D., McGraw, T. S. & Semple-Rowland, S. L. (2000). Comparative evaluation of cytokine profiles and reactive gliosis supports a critical role for interleukin-6 in neuron-glia signaling during regeneration. *J Neurosci Res*, 61(1), 10-20.

Streit, W. J. & Kreutzberg, G. W. (1987). Lectin binding by resting and reactive microglia. *J Neurocytol*, 16(2), 249-260.

Streit, W. J. & Kreutzberg, G. W. (1988). Response of endogenous glial cells to motor neuron degeneration induced by toxic ricin. *J Comp Neurol*, 268(2), 248-263.

Streit, W. J., Mrak, R. E. & Griffin, W. S. (2004a). Microglia and neuroinflammation: a pathological perspective. *J Neuroinflammation*, 1(1), 14.

Streit, W. J., Sammons, N. W., Kuhns, A. J. & Sparks, D. L. (2004b). Dystrophic microglia in the aging human brain. *Glia*, 45(2), 208-212.

Streit, W. J., Semple-Rowland, S. L., Hurley, S. D., Miller, R. C., Popovich, P. G. & Stokes, B. T. (1998). Cytokine mRNA profiles in contused spinal cord and axotomized facial nucleus suggest a beneficial role for inflammation and gliosis. *Exp Neurol*, 152(1), 74-87.

Streit, W. J. & Sparks, D. L. (1997). Activation of microglia in the brains of humans with heart disease and hypercholesterolemic rabbits. *J Mol Med*, 75(2), 130-138.

Streit, W. J., Walter, S. A. & Pennell, N. A. (1999). Reactive microgliosis. *Progress in Neurobiology*, 57, 563-581.

Stuesse, S. L., Cruce, W. L., Lovell, J. A., McBurney, D. L. & Crisp, T. (2000). Microglial proliferation in the spinal cord of aged rats with a sciatic nerve injury. *Neurosci Lett*, 287(2), 121-124.

Suh, H. S., Kim, M. O. & Lee, S. C. (2005). Inhibition of granulocyte-macrophage colony-stimulating factor signaling and microglial proliferation by anti-CD45RO: role of Hck tyrosine kinase and phosphatidylinositol 3-kinase/Akt. *J Immunol*, 174(5), 2712-2719.

Suzuki, Y., Claflin, J., Wang, X., Lengi, A. & Kikuchi, T. (2005). Microglia and macrophages as innate producers of interferon-gamma in the brain following infection with Toxoplasma gondii. *Int J Parasitol*, 35(1), 83-90.

Tonchev, A. B., Yamashima, T., Zhao, L. & Okano, H. (2003). Differential proliferative response in the postischemic hippocampus, temporal cortex, and olfactory bulb of young adult macaque monkeys. *Glia*, 42(3), 209-224.

van Rossum, D. & Hanisch, U. K. (2004). Microglia. *Metab Brain Dis*, 19(3-4), 393-411.

Watanabe, T., Yamamoto, T., Abe, Y., Saito, N., Kumagai, T. & Kayama, H. (1999). Differential activation of microglia after experimental spinal cord injury. *J Neurotrauma*, 16(3), 255-265.

Weldon, D. T., Rogers, S. D., Ghilardi, J. R., Finke, M. P., Cleary, J. P., O'Hare, E., Esler, W. P., Maggio, J. E. & Mantyh, P. W. (1998). Fibrillar beta-amyloid induces microglial phagocytosis, expression of inducible nitric oxide synthase, and loss of a select population of neurons in the rat CNS in vivo. *J Neurosci*, 18(6), 2161-2173.

Wierzba-Bobrowicz, T., Lewandowska, E., Kosno-Kruszewska, E., Lechowicz, W., Pasennik, E. & Schmidt-Sidor, B. (2004). Degeneration of microglial cells in frontal and temporal lobes of chronic schizophrenics. *Folia Neuropathol*, 42(3), 157-165.

Yang, L., Jones, N. R., Blumbergs, P. C., Van Den Heuvel, C., Moore, E. J., Manavis, J., Sarvestani, G. T. & Ghabriel, M. N. (2005). Severity-dependent expression of pro-inflammatory cytokines in traumatic spinal cord injury in the rat. *J Clin Neurosci*, 12(3), 276-284.

Ziaja, M. & Janeczko, K. (1999). Spatiotemporal patterns of microglial proliferation in rat brain injured at the postmitotic stage of postnatal development. *J Neurosci Res*, 58(3), 379-386.

In: Inflammation Research Perspectives
Editor: Giacomo T. Romano, pp. 61-79
ISBN: 978-1-60021-845-3

Chapter IV

NEUROTRAUMA AND INFLAMMATION

Roberta Brambilla, John R. Bethea and Valerie Bracchi-Ricard
The Miami Project To Cure Paralysis, Department of Neurological Surgery,
Miller School of Medicine, University of Miami, Miami, FL 33136, USA.

1. INTRODUCTION

Both traumatic brain injury (TBI) and spinal cord injury (SCI) are devastating conditions and leading causes of death and severe disability among young individuals. During the acute phase of injury, the primary mechanical impact to the brain or spinal cord induces an immediate tissue disruption causing focal hemorrhage, edema, release of excitatory amino acids and oxygen radicals. As a consequence of these initial events, a phase of secondary damage is initiated, during which neurochemical and metabolic alterations take place at the cellular level, ultimately leading to diffuse cell death and, often, tissue cavitation (in the spinal cord particularly, Hausmann, 2003). The inflammatory response is activated and the initial lesion expands as the injury progresses into a chronic phase. This inflammatory response is sustained by the concerted action of both peripheral cells (neutrophils, macrophages and lymphocytes) infiltrating the central nervous system (CNS) through a compromised blood brain barrier (BBB), and resident cells, particularly astrocytes and microglia. In these cell populations, which can be considered the resident inflammatory cells of the CNS, proinflammatory signal transduction cascades, such as the NF-κB pathway, are promptly activated following injury. This leads to the synthesis and release of cytokines, chemokines, extracellular matrix molecules, prostanoids, nitric oxide (NO), etc., which sustain and amplify the inflammatory reaction resulting in additional tissue loss.

The aim of this review is to discuss the contribution of glial cells to the inflammatory response of the CNS to neurotrauma, based on the vast body of data accumulated from *in vivo* models of TBI as well as SCI.

2. Post-Traumatic Inflammation in the Brain and Spinal Cord

2.1. Differences between Spinal Cord and Brain

Post-traumatic inflammation is a common feature of both TBI and SCI and contributes to the pathophysiology of these traumas. The initial mechanical injury to the brain or spinal cord initiates in both cases a complex cascade of events with common features like membrane disruption, hemorrhage, ischemia, vascular damage and both immediate (mostly necrotic) and delayed (apoptotic and necrotic) cell death. The secondary phase is characterized by a robust immune response with synthesis of cytokines and chemokines, coordinated infiltration of the injury site by peripheral leukocytes, activation of resident immune cells (microglia) resulting acutely in the clearance of cell debris but chronically in bystander cell damage and progressive tissue loss. The final lesion site is far greater than that observed few hours post-injury. Schnell and colleagues provided evidence that the acute inflammatory response to traumatic injury is significantly greater in the spinal cord than the cerebral cortex using the same mouse strain with similar incision lesions performed in the frontal cortex and spinal cord (Schnell et al., 1999). The number of neutrophils recruited at the lesion 1 day following injury was much greater in the spinal cord than in the brain. This was correlated with a greater upregulation of intercellular adhesion molecules, in particular the platelet-endothelial cell adhesion molecule (PECAM) in the spinal cord. In addition, whereas neutrophils were closely lining the lesion sites in the cortex, the distribution in the spinal cord was more widespread. Similarly, the macrophages/microglia reaction was also considerably greater in the spinal cord. Lymphocytes were recruited at a relatively low number in these paradigms, but again in contrast with the brain, they could be found as far as 3-4 mm from the lesion. The astrocytic response to trauma, as measured by GFAP upregulation, was more pronounced in the spinal cord at 1 day post-injury, and doubled that of the forebrain at 2 days. Correlating with the neutrophil recruitment profile, the area of BBB breakdown, as revealed by horseradish peroxidase extravasation, was two to three times larger in the spinal cord and lasted up to 14 days (last time point studied) whereas in the brain the BBB was reestablished after 10 days.

2.2. Differences between Mouse and Rat

The study by Schnell and colleagues was carried out in a mouse model. Although mice are very useful especially to study gene-specific function (knockout and transgenic mice models) they also display a unique pathology following spinal cord contusion, which is the result of a distinct inflammatory response (Sroga et al., 2003). One major difference between mice and other mammals (rats, cats, monkeys, humans) is the absence of fluid-filled cystic cavities in mice after SCI. Instead, the lesion site is filled with dense fibrous connective tissue. Sroga and colleagues reported differences in the distribution, magnitude, and composition of the inflammatory response to SCI between Lewis rats and C57BL/6 mice (Sroga et al., 2003). A major difference was the significant infiltration of T-cells and dendritic cells in the rat contused spinal cord. The time-course of macrophages/microglia activation was similar between rat and mouse. The role of microglia/macrophages remains controversial as they can produce a number of inflammatory cytokines, chemokines, but also growth-promoting factors. Differences in the mediators released by mouse or rat macrophages/microglia could result in a species-specific post-injury cellular environment (Sroga et al., 2003).

2.3. Strain Differences

Differences have also been reported between strains of rats following SCI, where contused Lewis rats had an elevated microglia/macrophages response and an early infiltration of T-cells compared to Sprague-Dawley rats (Popovich et al., 1997). Mice also exhibit differences, some strains being excitotoxic-resistant and others sensitive. Enhanced cellular repair and axonal growth was observed in 129X1/SvJ mice, which have diminished chronic inflammatory response compared to C57Bl/6 mice receiving identical contusion to the spinal cord (Ma et al., 2004).

2.4. Gender

The inflammatory response to brain trauma may be affected by hormone levels. This issue is not well addressed and most *in vivo* SCI and TBI studies are conducted in male rats (to avoid hormonal issues) or female mice (because of frequent urinary tract infections in male mice after SCI). However, evidence is accumulating that the response to trauma, and particularly the inflammatory response, may be affected by the gender. Less inflammatory cells infiltrating the lesion were observed in female C57Bl/6 mice compared to males after SCI (Farooque et al., 2005). Similarly, in rats after head injury females displayed a higher survival rate and smaller lesion size than males (Roof and Hall, 2000; Bramlett and Dietrich, 2001). In contrast, in a controlled-cortical impact model no differences were observed between genders (Hall et al., 2005).

2.5. Age

Enhanced glial activation was observed in aged (36 months) compared to young (3 months) rats following cortical stab injury (Kyrkanides et al., 2001). This was correlated with a greater increase in tumor necrosis factor (TNF), interleukin-6 (IL-6), interleukin-1β (IL-1β) in aged rats at 6 hours post-injury, decreasing at 72 hours to levels similar to young rats. In addition, significant increase in inducible nitric oxide synthase (iNOS), intercellular adhesion molecule (ICAM) and matrix metalloproteinase-9 (MMP-9) was observed in aged rats and still remained sustained at 72 hours, whereas in young rats the levels had returned to that of sham controls. Clinical studies have established that the outcome following TBI is worsened by age.

3. NF-κB Activation Following Trauma

The transcription factor nuclear factor kappa-B (NF-κB) regulates the expression of many genes encoding cytokines, chemokines, inflammatory enzymes (cyclooxygenase and nitric oxide synthase), and mediating the inflammatory responses in the CNS. Following TBI and SCI NF-κB is rapidly activated in the brain (Yang et al., 1995; Nonaka et al., 1999; Nomoto et al., 2001; Sanz et al., 2002; Lotocki et al., 2004) and spinal cord (Bethea et al., 1998; Kim et al., 2001; Conti et al., 2003; La Rosa et al., 2004; Brambilla et al., 2005; Genovese et al., 2005).

NF-κB activation has been reported to occur in various cell types including neurons, astrocytes, microglia/macrophages, and oligodendrocytes (Bethea et al., 1998; Nonaka et al., 1999; Nomoto et al., 2001; Sanz et al., 2002; Yune et al., 2004), using coimmunolocalization of an activated form of p65 with cell-specific markers. The spatio-temporal activation of NF-κB varies with the type of injury, the animal model and the CNS compartment.

In a parasagittal fluid percussion model of TBI in the rat, NF-κB was first found to be activated mostly in injured axons of the cerebral cortex, within 24 hours in microglia/macrophages and within 48 hours in astrocytes (Nonaka et al., 1999). Interestingly, NF-κB activation persisted in microglia/macrophages and astrocytes up to 1 year following trauma at the margin of the progressively enlarging necrotic cavities, which correspond also to the regions undergoing persistent tissue loss. These observations suggest a role for astrocytes and microglia/macrophages in the prolonged inflammatory process through sustained activation of NF-κB. In a different model of brain injury consisting in the thermal ablation of a portion of the cortex in mice, a delayed activation of NF-κB was observed (Nomoto et al., 2001). Indeed, the first weak p65 nuclear immunoreactivity was observed 2 days after injury in mononuclear cells surrounding the lesion. Later, at 4 and 8 days, a strong p65 immunostaining was found in astrocytes and macrophage/microglia around the lesion. This NF-κB activation faded by 14 days and was absent at 28 days. Different patterns of activation were also observed in the lesioned immature rat brain, which is more plastic than the adult brain with ameboid microglia present under physiological conditions (Sanz et al., 2002). In this model of cortical aspiration the glial response was very rapid with microglia reactivity observed at 4 hours post-lesion within the neurodegenerative area bordering the cavity, and reactive hypertrophic astrocyte response evident at 10 hours in the damaged cortex. NF-κB activation was observed not only in hypertrophic reactive astrocytes surrounding the lesion and forming the glial scar, but also in white matter astrocytes located at deeper levels into the brain parenchyma (e.g., corpus callosum) (Sanz et al., 2002). In contrast to the long-lasting microglial NF-κB activation reported in adult brain (Nonaka et al., 1999), the injury to the post-natal rat brain induced a pulse-like activation of microglial NF-κB. In this study by Sanz and colleagues the latest time point was 7 days post-injury. In summary, those studies agree on an initial activation of NF-κB in microglial cells followed by activation in astrocytes in areas of progressive tissue damage, strongly suggesting a role for glial cells and the NF-κB pathway in the secondary injury process.

In a model of spinal cord contusion in the adult rat, Bethea and colleagues reported the presence of activated NF-κB in macrophages/microglia and endothelial cells starting 30 minutes post-injury and lasting for 72 hours, which was the last time point studied. Activated

NF-κB appeared in neurons at 24 hours post-injury. Although no p65 immunostaining was observed in astrocytes up to 72 hours post-injury, it is possible that delayed astroglial reactivity would have been observed at later time points. In fact, a more recent study using a transgenic mouse model where NF-κB was selectively blocked in astrocytes clearly implicated astroglial cells and the NF-κB pathway in the pathophysiology of SCI (Brambilla et al., 2005). Immediately after injury (1 hour), NF-κB was primarily activated in astrocytes and the events initiated thereafter lead to the loss of locomotor function, as transgenic mice with inactive NF-κB in astrocytes recovered from contusion-induced hindlimb paralysis significantly better than wild type mice. This appeared to be due to the reduced expression of NF-κB-dependent proinflammatory chemokines interferon-inducible protein-10 (IP10) and monocyte chemoattractant protein-1 (MCP-1) in astrocytes, as well as of the proteoglycans neurocan and phosphacan, which are synthesized by astrocytes and take part in the formation of the glial scar.

The chronic activation of NF-κB in astrocytes and/or microglia/macrophages indicates the importance of these cells in the maintenance of the inflammatory response after injury, which appears to be associated with the progressive loss of nervous tissue and concomitant loss of neurological functions. In support of these observations is the use of various pharmacological strategies aimed at reducing the inflammatory response that improve the functional outcome after trauma and inhibit NF-κB activation (Xu et al., 1998; La Rosa et al., 2004; Ravikumar et al., 2004; Genovese et al., 2005). Although it is tempting to view NF-κB as a foe, we need to keep in mind that NF-κB does regulate not only the expression of proinflammatory molecules but also of anti-apoptotic factors like cIAP2 (Kim et al., 2001) and antioxidative enzymes like manganese superoxide dismutase (MnSOD) (Yune et al., 2004). Furthermore, other transcription factors may be playing important roles either on their own or in concert with NF-κB.

4. Cytokine Production

Following trauma to the CNS cytokine levels rapidly increase at the site of lesion. Although several members of the cytokine family have well demonstrated anti-inflammatory properties, overall these molecules are considered amongst the principal mediators of the inflammatory response (see for review Brambilla et al., 2005). Cytokines are produced at high concentrations not only by infiltrating immune cells, but also by resident microglia and astrocytes in the CNS parenchyma, particularly during the early phase of injury. A correlation between the severity of the injury and the levels of proinflammatory cytokines was established (Yang et al., 2005).

4.1. TNFα

Reactive astrocytes at the lesion site begin synthesizing TNFα within minutes (Kita et al., 2000; Lee et al., 2000) and appear to keep up the production for a relatively narrow window of time (Bartholdi and Schwab, 1997; Streit et al., 1998; Yan et al., 1999; Yan et al., 2001).

At later times the astrocytic production of TNFα is sustained by cells surrounding the lesion (glial scar) or at even farther distances from the site of damage (Kita et al., 2000). This initial burst of TNFα is believed to be a further signal for the production of more proinflammatory cytokines from the glial cells (not only astrocytes, but also microglia) and from infiltrating leukocytes entering the CNS, therefore acting as a major player in the amplification of the inflammatory response (Pan et al., 2002). The early inhibition of TNFα and TNFα signaling after trauma, in fact, has generally proven to be neuroprotective and is paralleled by the reduction in the expression of other proinflammatory molecules. As an example, the topical application of TNF antiserum at the site of injury significantly attenuated swelling, edema, disturbances of the microvascular permeability and cell injury induced by SCI (Sharma et al., 2003). TNF antiserum also diminished the SCI-induced upregulation of neuronal nitric oxide synthase (nNOS), indicating a possible beneficial role in preventing NO-mediated oxidative damage following injury.

Two other members of the TNF superfamily of cytokines, Fas and FasL (also called CD95 and CD95L, or APO-1 and APO-1L), have also been implicated in the inflammatory response triggered following CNS trauma. Both molecules are upregulated at various degrees in neurons, astrocytes, oligodendrocytes and microglia following TBI and SCI (Beer et al., 2000; Casha et al., 2001; Zurita et al., 2001; Qiu et al., 2002; Demjen et al., 2004) and act as proinflammatory and proapoptotic signals by activating the NF-κB pathway (see for review Wajant et al., 2003; Dosreis et al., 2004). In astrocytes Fas ligation (permanent death receptor activation) induces the upregulation of cytokines and chemokines such as IL-6, MCP-1 and IL-8 (Saas et al., 1999; Lee et al., 2000), which can propagate the inflammatory response by stimulating blood cell chemotaxis into the injured CNS, potentially preventing functional recovery. On the other hand, neutralization of FasL by administration of a FasL-specific antibody lead to increased oligodendrocyte and neuronal survival, axonal regeneration and improved functional outcome following SCI (Demjen et al., 2004).

4.2. IL-6

In the CNS IL-6 production, which originates largely from astrocytes and microglial cells, is upregulated following injury. Although a number of neuroprotective effects are attributed to this molecule (Morganti-Kossmann et al., 2002), a great body of evidence demonstrates the proinflammatory properties of IL-6, implicating it in the development of secondary tissue damage after trauma (see for review John et al., 2003; Brambilla et al., 2005). The destructive potential of deregulated IL-6 is evident from studies by Campbell and colleagues (Campbell et al., 1993; Barnum et al., 1996) showing that transgenic mice overexpressing IL-6 in astrocytes display extensive brain damage (neurodegeneration, BBB disruption, learning deficit) caused by a persistent state of inflammation. This is supported by studies in IL-6 knockout mice, which exhibit reduced inflammation and depressed astrogliosis after focal cryo-injury compared to wild type mice (Penkowa et al., 1999). Furthermore, in models of SCI, blocking the IL-6 receptor or IL-6 bioactivity with specific neutralizing antibodies suppressed reactive astrogliosis, decreased scar tissue formation, immune cell infiltration, iNOS activity and secondary damage, leading to significant improvement of functional recovery (Tuna et al., 2001; Okada et al., 2004). Along the same line, administration of a bioactive IL-6/soluble IL-6 receptor fusion protein (H-IL-6), secreted by genetically engineered fibroblasts grafted at the site of lesion, induced amplification of the inflammatory response resulting in increased neutrophil infiltration and consequent elevation in reactive oxygen species (Lacroix et al., 2002).

Like IL-6, leukemia inhibitory factor (LIF) plays a key role in inflammation and can act in both a pro- and anti-inflammatory fashion (see for review Gadient and Patterson, 1999). While LIF has been extensively studied in a number of inflammatory conditions (e.g., rheumatoid arthritis), few studies have investigated the role of LIF in traumatic injury to the CNS. As indicated in a stab wound injury model of CNS trauma, LIF expression is rapidly upregulated predominantly in astrocytes in the lesion penumbra (Banner et al., 1997). In this context, LIF appears to operate as a proinflammatory signal by recruiting peripheral monocytes and inducing reactive gliosis (Sugiura et al., 2000).

4.3. IL-1β

IL-1β is expressed at low levels by neurons and glial cells under physiological conditions and like TNF is quickly upregulated within the CNS parenchyma following trauma. Studies agree on a robust and transient increase in IL-1β mRNA as early as 1 hour post-injury in both TBI (Fan et al., 1995; Rostworowski et al., 1997; Herx et al., 2000) and SCI models (Bartholdi and Schwab, 1997; Wang et al., 1997; Streit et al., 1998; Pan et al., 2002). Increase in IL-1β protein levels (measured by ELISA) is detected as soon as 1 to 4 hours following injury to the spinal cord or brain (Wang et al., 1997; Knoblach and Faden, 2000; Ciallella et al., 2002; Kinoshita et al., 2002). In a rat spinal cord contusion model, IL-1βprotein levels were sustained until 72 hours post-injury and remained elevated for 1 week (Wang et al., 1997), whereas in the brain IL-1β levels returned to baseline by 24-72 hours following trauma (Knoblach and Faden, 2000; Ciallella et al., 2002; Kinoshita et al., 2002). This would suggest a stronger inflammation in the spinal cord. IL-1β, which is mainly produced by microglia in the injured CNS (Woodroofe et al., 1991; Bartholdi and Schwab, 1997) contributes to the disruption of the BBB, stimulates astrogliosis and glial scar formation, and is involved in neuronal damage. In fact, intracerebral microinjection of IL-1β in rats induced a transient inflammatory reaction accompanied by apoptotic cell death (Holmin and Mathiesen, 2000). In a spinal cord contusion model in rats, IL-1β was implicated in the induction of apoptosis in neurons and oligodendrocytes through caspase-3 activation (Nesic et al., 2001). Recently the p38/mitogen-activated protein kinase (p38/MAPK) pathway was involved in mediating IL-1β-induced neuronal apoptosis (Wang et al., 2005). Furthermore, infusion of IL-1 receptor antagonist (IL-1ra) for 72 hours in the injured spinal cord using an osmotic minipump completely abolished the increase in contusion-induced apoptosis as well as the caspase activity (Nesic et al., 2001). Similarly, injections of IL-1ra in the contused brain starting at 15 minutes and up to 48 hours following injury resulted in reduced damage 3 and 7 days later (Toulmond and Rothwell, 1995). Likewise, transgenic mice overexpressing IL-1ra in astrocytes also displayed a higher neurological recovery following closed head injury compared to wild type mice (Tehranian et al., 2002). In contrast, in a rat brain contusion model, intracerebroventricular administration of IL-1ra or soluble IL-1 receptor type I starting at 15 minutes and until 8 hours after injury, did not significantly improve neurological outcome as assessed by a series of motor tasks performed at 1, 7 and 14 days post-injury (Knoblach and Faden, 2000). The discrepancies between the studies may be explained by the different times of treatment. IL-1β like other proinflammatory cytokines does not have only deleterious effects. It also promotes angiogenesis, wound healing and plasticity. Injecting recombinant IL-1β into the dorsal column of the spinal cord undergoing Wallerian degeneration triggered rapid macrophage/microglial activation and myelin clearance (Perrin et al., 2005). Increased IL-1β levels following brain injury were linked to increased levels of ciliary neurotrophic factor (CNTF), an important survival factor for neurons and maturation factor for oligodendrocytes (Herx et al., 2000). Upregulation of IL-1β following TBI was also temporally followed by an increase in nerve growth factor (NGF), which was suppressed by IL-1ra (DeKosky et al., 1996). Similarly, hypothermia decreased IL-1β and NGF expression (Goss et al., 1995).

4.4. TGFβ

Various members of the transforming growth factor beta (TGFβ) family of cytokines have been implicated in the pathophysiology of CNS injury. As many other cytokines, TGFβ has both anti-inflammatory and proinflammatory/profibrotic properties that can lead to either beneficial (e.g., reduction of cytokine production) or detrimental (scar formation) effects following injury (Chin et al., 2004). As a fibrotic molecule (Ihn, 2002), TGFβis mainly produced by astrocytes, where it induces the synthesis of extracellular matrix molecules and proteoglycans (Westergren-Thorsson et al., 1992; Lagord et al., 2002), which are major constituents of the glial scar and inhibitory to axon regeneration. Following SCI, both TGFβ1 and TGFβ2 are upregulated (Lagord et al., 2002; Brambilla et al., 2005), but it is the expression of TGFβ2, rather than TGFβ1, that apparently correlates with the deposition of the glial scar (Lagord et al., 2002). Treatments aimed at inhibiting TGFβ biological activity (e.g. neutralizing antibodies) have been successful at reducing the deposition of scar tissue (Logan et al., 1994; Moon and Fawcett, 2001) establishing an environment more suitable for axonal regeneration. Interestingly, a recent work from our group has indicated that the early expression of TGFβ2 induced by SCI is significantly reduced in transgenic mice where NF-κB is selectively inhibited in astrocytes, and so is the expression of the scar forming proteoglycans neurocan and phosphacan. This demonstrates that TGFβ2 production occurs primarily in astrocytes following SCI and is transcriptionally dependent on NF-κB. The inhibition of this very important proinflammatory pathway in this cells type prevents TGFβ2 expression and results in reduced scar formation and improved functional outcome (Brambilla et al., 2005).

4.5. EMAPII

The endothelial monocyte-activating polypeptide II (EMAPII) is an antiangiogenic and proinflammatory cytokine expressed by microglia/macrophages (Schluesener et al., 1997). In both a rat spinal cord transection model (Mueller et al., 2003a) and a rat cortical stab wound injury model (Mueller et al., 2003b), a significant increase in the number of EMAPII$^+$ microglia/macrophages was observed at the lesion site peaking at 3 and 5 days following SCI and TBI, respectively. In both injury paradigms the EMAPII immunoreactivity declined gradually over several weeks, but still remained elevated compared to sham-operated animals, especially in the SCI model. Clusters of EMAPII$^+$ macrophages/microglia were observed in Virchow-Robin spaces in both the brain and spinal cord. EMAPII might contribute to the formation of edema by compromising the blood flow through its ability to activate P- and E-selectin-mediated platelet and leukocyte rolling on endothelium. The prolonged accumulation of EMAPII$^+$ macrophages/microglia in regions of neuronal death at the lesion site suggests a role for this proinflammatory cytokine in the secondary damage following TBI and SCI.

5. Chemokines

Chemokines are small pleiotropic molecules that act as signals not only for the recruitment of inflammatory leukocytes to the CNS but also for the activation of resident cells of the CNS (e.g., microglia and astrocytes) which, as well as leukocytes, express chemokine receptors (Cartier et al., 2005). In addition, members of the CXC group of chemokines are regulators of angiogenesis, acting either as angiogenic or angiostatic factors (Bernardini et al., 2003). In CNS trauma and other neurodegenerative disorders chemokines (e.g., CXCL10/IP10, CCL2/MCP1, CCL3/MIP1α, CCL5/RANTES), which are produced primarily in astrocytes and, in some cases, in microglial cells, are highly upregulated (Ransohoff et al., 1993; Lee et al., 2000; Otto et al., 2001; Babcock et al., 2003; Baron et al., 2005; Brambilla et al., 2005). CXCL10/IP10, CCL2/MCP1 and CCL5/RANTES expression peaks within 1 day after SCI (Lee et al., 2000; Ravikumar et al., 2004; Brambilla et al., 2005) and treatments resulting in reduction of their production have proven to be neuroprotective. Infusion of the broad spectrum chemokine antagonist vMIPII after SCI diminished hematogenous infiltration and axonal degeneration (Ghirnikar et al., 2001). Similarly, inhibition of astroglial NF-κB in a transgenic mouse model resulted in reduced CXCL10/IP10 and CCL2/MCP1 expression following SCI and improved functional outcome (Brambilla et al., 2005). Antibody neutralization of CXCL10/IP10 beginning 1 day prior to hemisection injury significantly reduced the infiltration of T-lymphocytes into the spinal cord parenchyma, limiting tissue loss and functional deficit (Gonzalez et al., 2003). In a separate study, Glaser and colleagues demonstrated that anti-CXCL10/IP10 treatment of SCI improved blood flow and oxygen supply to the injury by counteracting the angiostatic properties of CXCL10/IP10, hence promoting angiogenesis and ultimately ameliorating the functional outcome (Glaser et al., 2004).

In an entorhinal cortex brain injury model, CXCL10 was expressed by lesioned neurons (Rappert et al., 2004). In this model of anterograde (Wallerian) axonal degeneration, microglial cells expressing the receptor for CXCL10, namely CXCR3, were attracted to the damaged axons expressing the chemokine. Conversely, in the CXCR3 knockout mice there was a lack of recruitment of microglial cells and maintenance of denervated dendrites. Whether this preservation of dendrites is functionally relevant or not remains to be determined.

6. Oxy-Radical Generating Enzymes

6.1. Nitric Oxide Synthase

Nitric oxide (NO) and reactive oxygen species exert multiple modulating effects on inflammation and regulation of immune responses. Low concentrations of NO produced by constitutive and neuronal nitric oxide synthases (cNOS, nNOS) inhibit adhesion molecule expression, cytokine and chemokine synthesis and leukocyte adhesion and transmigration. Conversely, large amounts of NO, generated primarily by inducible nitric oxide synthase (iNOS/NOS-2), can be cytotoxic and proinflammatory. NO produced after injury by iNOS in activated glia (both astroglia and microglia/macrophages) has been associated with neuronal cell death and functional impairment following CNS injury. Indeed, in many studies, treatments with various iNOS inhibitors (aminoguanidines, 1400W, antisense oligonucleotides) resulted in reduced apoptotic and necrotic cell death of neurons and improved functional outcome following TBI (Chatzipanteli et al., 1999; Jafarian-Tehrani et al., 2005) and SCI (Chatzipanteli et al., 2002; Pearse et al., 2003; Kwak et al., 2005). On the other hand, the prolonged treatment with aminoguanidine was also shown to have deleterious effects in a rat model of TBI with a significant decrease in the number of surviving hippocampal neurons 21 days after injury, suggesting that iNOS may have some protective functions (Sinz et al., 1999). The proinflammatory and deleterious role of NO generated through iNOS was demonstrated in recent studies conducted in iNOS knockout mice. In both a SCI (extradural compression of the thoracic spinal cord, Isaksson et al., 2005) and a TBI (severe aseptic cryogenic cerebral injury, Jones et al., 2004) model, iNOS knockout mice showed significantly improved functional outcome accompanied by reduced lesion volume compared to wild type littermates. In contrast, a recent study by Bayir and colleagues reported an enhanced oxidative stress in iNOS-deficient mice after controlled cortical impact, which would imply a neuroprotective role for iNOS (Bayir et al., 2005). However, in this study the authors did not provide any behavioral outcome measures.

6.2 Cyclooxygenases

The production of pronociceptive and proinflammatory prostaglandins is dependent on the activity of cyclooxygenases (COXs). Two COX enzymes have been identified: a constitutively expressed COX-1 and an inducible highly regulated COX-2 (Minghetti and

Levi, 1998; Vanegas and Schaible, 2001). Interestingly, while COX-2 is hardly expressed in most tissues under physiological conditions, it is detected at significant levels in the brain (Seibert et al., 1994). By immnunohistochemistry, COX-2 was found in both brain and spinal cord neurons, and in spinal cord white matter astrocytes (Beiche et al., 1998). The difference between brain and spinal cord astrocytes was also observed *in vitro* where spinal cord but not cortical astrocytes released prostaglandins when stimulated with substance P (Marriott et al., 1991). COX-2 mRNA and protein are quickly upregulated within hours following both TBI (Dash et al., 2000; Strauss et al., 2000; Cernak et al., 2001; Kunz et al., 2002) and SCI (Resnick et al., 1998; Adachi et al., 2005). The temporal expression profiles vary depending on the model and the severity of the injury but all studies concur that COX-2 protein levels are sustained for several days following injury. In a lateral cortical impact model, COX-2 protein levels peaked 1-3 days post-injury and returned to sham levels by 7 days (Strauss et al., 2000). In contrast, in an impact acceleration model, which has diffuse axonal injury as a major component, COX-2 remained elevated at least for 12 days post-injury (Cernak et al., 2001). The cell type which expresses COX-2 after trauma is controversial. Following TBI, COX-2 immunoreactivity was found in neurons (Dash et al., 2000; Strauss et al., 2000) and glial cells around the injury (Strauss et al., 2000). Following SCI, COX-2 was localized to endothelial cells lining blood vessels but was not observed in neurons, astrocytes, or macrophage/microglia (Adachi et al., 2005). However, following intraparenchymal injection of IL-1β in the spinal cord, Tonai and colleagues could detect COX-2 in glial cells, leukocytes and vascular endothelial cells (Tonai et al., 1999). Similar intraparenchymal administration of IL-1β in the brain induced COX-2 expression (Moore et al., 2004). COX-1, which has been less studied than COX-2, appears to be predominantly expressed by macrophages/microglia after both TBI and SCI (Mueller et al., 2003a, b). Pharmacological treatments with non steroidal anti-inflammatory drugs aimed at inhibiting COX-2 activity have proven efficacious in reducing the inflammatory response following trauma and improving the functional outcome both in SCI and TBI models (Resnick et al., 1998; Cernak et al., 2001; Hains et al., 2001; Hurley et al., 2002; Gopez et al., 2005).

7. Conclusion

Inflammation contributes significantly to the secondary injury mechanisms that follow both traumatic brain and spinal cord injuries, with resident astrocytes and microglia as major players by releasing proinflammatory cytokines, chemokines, NO, prostaglandins, etc. If inflammation is a common factor to traumatic injury, its development varies depending on a number of factors including CNS compartment (brain or spinal cord), type of injury (focal or diffuse), age, gender, and genetic background. Interestingly, many of these factors can be associated with differences in astrocyte and microglia reactivity. These differences are crucial as they may affect the window during which an anti-inflammatory treatment strategy would be the most beneficial. As reported in many studies, the same cytokines that are proinflammatory early following injury also play beneficial roles later during regeneration.

ACKNOWLEDGEMENTS

This work was supported by National Insitute of Health grants NS37130 and NS051709 (both to JR Bethea) and by the Miami Project to Cure Paralysis.

REFERENCES

Adachi K, Yimin Y, Satake K, Matsuyama Y, Ishiguro N, Sawada M, Hirata Y, Kiuchi K (2005) Localization of cyclooxygenase-2 induced following traumatic spinal cord injury. *Neurosci Res 51*:73-80.

Babcock AA, Kuziel WA, Rivest S, Owens T (2003) Chemokine expression by glial cells directs leukocytes to sites of axonal injury in the CNS. *J Neurosci 23*:7922-7930.

Banner LR, Moayeri NN, Patterson PH (1997) Leukemia inhibitory factor is expressed in astrocytes following cortical brain injury. *Exp Neurol 147*:1-9.

Barnum SR, Jones JL, Muller-Ladner U, Samimi A, Campbell IL (1996) Chronic complement C3 gene expression in the CNS of transgenic mice with astrocyte-targeted interleukin-6 expression. *Glia 18*:107-117.

Baron P, Bussini S, Cardin V, Corbo M, Conti G, Galimberti D, Scarpini E, Bresolin N, Wharton SB, Shaw PJ, Silani V (2005) Production of monocyte chemoattractant protein-1 in amyotrophic lateral sclerosis. *Muscle Nerve 32*:541-544.

Bartholdi D, Schwab ME (1997) Expression of pro-inflammatory cytokine and chemokine mRNA upon experimental spinal cord injury in mouse: an in situ hybridization study. *Eur J Neurosci 9*:1422-1438.

Bayir H, Kagan VE, Borisenko GG, Tyurina YY, Janesko KL, Vagni VA, Billiar TR, Williams DL, Kochanek PM (2005) Enhanced oxidative stress in iNOS-deficient mice after traumatic brain injury: support for a neuroprotective role of iNOS. *J Cereb Blood Flow Metab 25*:673-684.

Beer R, Franz G, Schopf M, Reindl M, Zelger B, Schmutzhard E, Poewe W, Kampfl A (2000) Expression of Fas and Fas ligand after experimental traumatic brain injury in the rat. *J Cereb Blood Flow Metab 20*:669-677.

Beiche F, Klein T, Nusing R, Neuhuber W, Goppelt-Struebe M (1998) Localization of cyclooxygenase-2 and prostaglandin E2 receptor EP3 in the rat lumbar spinal cord. *J Neuroimmunol 89*:26-34.

Bernardini G, Ribatti D, Spinetti G, Morbidelli L, Ziche M, Santoni A, Capogrossi MC, Napolitano M (2003) Analysis of the role of chemokines in angiogenesis. *J Immunol* Methods *273*:83-101.

Bethea JR, Castro M, Keane RW, Lee TT, Dietrich WD, Yezierski RP (1998) Traumatic spinal cord injury induces nuclear factor-kappaB activation. *J Neurosci 18*:3251-3260.

Brambilla R, Bracchi-Ricard V, Hu WH, Frydel B, Bramwell A, Karmally S, Green EJ, Bethea JR (2005) Inhibition of astroglial nuclear factor kappaB reduces inflammation and improves functional recovery after spinal cord injury. *J Exp Med 202*:145-156.

Brambilla R, Bracchi-Ricard V, Bethea, JR (2005) Cytokines in brain trauma and spinal cord injury. In: *Cytokines and the CNS.* Taylor & Francis Group, Boca Raton, pp 299-326.

Bramlett HM, Dietrich WD (2001) Neuropathological protection after traumatic brain injury in intact female rats versus males or ovariectomized females. *J Neurotrauma* 18:891-900.

Campbell IL, Abraham CR, Masliah E, Kemper P, Inglis JD, Oldstone MB, Mucke L (1993) Neurologic disease induced in transgenic mice by cerebral overexpression of interleukin 6. *Proc Natl Acad Sci U S A 90*:10061-10065.

Cartier L, Hartley O, Dubois-Dauphin M, Krause KH (2005) Chemokine receptors in the central nervous system: role in brain inflammation and neurodegenerative diseases. *Brain Res Brain Res Rev 48*:16-42.

Casha S, Yu WR, Fehlings MG (2001) Oligodendroglial apoptosis occurs along degenerating axons and is associated with FAS and p75 expression following spinal cord injury in the rat. *Neuroscience 103*:203-218.

Cernak I, O'Connor C, Vink R (2001) Activation of cyclo-oxygenase-2 contributes to motor and cognitive dysfunction following diffuse traumatic brain injury in rats. *Clin Exp Pharmacol Physiol 28*:922-925.

Chatzipanteli K, Wada K, Busto R, Dietrich WD (1999) Effects of moderate hypothermia on constitutive and inducible nitric oxide synthase activities after traumatic brain injury in the rat. *J Neurochem 72*:2047-2052.

Chatzipanteli K, Garcia R, Marcillo AE, Loor KE, Kraydieh S, Dietrich WD (2002) Temporal and segmental distribution of constitutive and inducible nitric oxide synthases after traumatic spinal cord injury: effect of aminoguanidine treatment. *J Neurotrauma 19*:639-651.

Chin D, Boyle GM, Parsons PG, Coman WB (2004) What is transforming growth factor-beta (TGF-beta)? *Br J Plast Surg 57*:215-221.

Ciallella JR, Ikonomovic MD, Paljug WR, Wilbur YI, Dixon CE, Kochanek PM, Marion DW, DeKosky ST (2002) Changes in expression of amyloid precursor protein and interleukin-1beta after experimental traumatic brain injury in rats. *J Neurotrauma 19*:1555-1567.

Conti A, Cardali S, Genovese T, Di Paola R, La Rosa G (2003) Role of inflammation in the secondary injury following experimental spinal cord trauma. *J Neurosurg Sci 47*:89-94.

Dash PK, Mach SA, Moore AN (2000) Regional expression and role of cyclooxygenase-2 following experimental traumatic brain injury. *J Neurotrauma 17*:69-81.

DeKosky ST, Styren SD, O'Malley ME, Goss JR, Kochanek P, Marion D, Evans CH, Robbins PD (1996) Interleukin-1 receptor antagonist suppresses neurotrophin response in injured rat brain. *Ann Neurol 39*:123-127.

Demjen D, Klussmann S, Kleber S, Zuliani C, Stieltjes B, Metzger C, Hirt UA, Walczak H, Falk W, Essig M, Edler L, Krammer PH, Martin-Villalba A (2004) Neutralization of CD95 ligand promotes regeneration and functional recovery after spinal cord injury. *Nat Med 10*:389-395.

Dosreis GA, Borges VM, Zin WA (2004) The central role of Fas-ligand cell signaling in inflammatory lung diseases. *J Cell Mol Med 8*:285-293.

Fan L, Young PR, Barone FC, Feuerstein GZ, Smith DH, McIntosh TK (1995) Experimental brain injury induces expression of interleukin-1 beta mRNA in the rat brain. *Brain Res Mol Brain Res 30*:125-130.

Farooque M, Suo Z, Arnold PM, Wulser MJ, Chou CT, Vancura RW, Fowler S, Festoff BW (2005) Gender-related differences in recovery of locomotor function after spinal cord injury in mice. *Spinal Cord.*

Gadient RA, Patterson PH (1999) Leukemia inhibitory factor, Interleukin 6, and other cytokines using the GP130 transducing receptor: roles in inflammation and injury. *Stem Cells 17*:127-137.

Genovese T, Mazzon E, Muia C, Patel NS, Threadgill MD, Bramanti P, De Sarro A, Thiemermann C, Cuzzocrea S (2005) Inhibitors of poly(ADP-ribose) polymerase modulate signal transduction pathways and secondary damage in experimental spinal cord trauma. *J Pharmacol Exp Ther 312*:449-457.

Ghirnikar RS, Lee YL, Eng LF (2001) Chemokine antagonist infusion promotes axonal sparing after spinal cord contusion injury in rat. *J Neurosci Res 64*:582-589.

Glaser J, Gonzalez R, Perreau VM, Cotman CW, Keirstead HS (2004) Neutralization of the chemokine CXCL10 enhances tissue sparing and angiogenesis following spinal cord injury. *J Neurosci Res 77*:701-708.

Gonzalez R, Glaser J, Liu MT, Lane TE, Keirstead HS (2003) Reducing inflammation decreases secondary degeneration and functional deficit after spinal cord injury. *Exp Neurol 184*:456-463.

Gopez JJ, Yue H, Vasudevan R, Malik AS, Fogelsanger LN, Lewis S, Panikashvili D, Shohami E, Jansen SA, Narayan RK, Strauss KI (2005) Cyclooxygenase-2-specific inhibitor improves functional outcomes, provides neuroprotection, and reduces inflammation in a rat model of traumatic brain injury. *Neurosurgery 56*:590-604.

Goss JR, Styren SD, Miller PD, Kochanek PM, Palmer AM, Marion DW, DeKosky ST (1995) Hypothermia attenuates the normal increase in interleukin 1 beta RNA and nerve growth factor following traumatic brain injury in the rat. *J Neurotrauma 12*:159-167.

Hains BC, Yucra JA, Hulsebosch CE (2001) Reduction of pathological and behavioral deficits following spinal cord contusion injury with the selective cyclooxygenase-2 inhibitor NS-398. *J Neurotrauma 18*:409-423.

Hall ED, Gibson TR, Pavel KM (2005) Lack of a gender difference in post-traumatic neurodegeneration in the mouse controlled cortical impact injury model. *J Neurotrauma 22*:669-679.

Hausmann ON (2003) Post-traumatic inflammation following spinal cord injury. *Spinal Cord 41*:369-378.

Herx LM, Rivest S, Yong VW (2000) Central nervous system-initiated inflammation and neurotrophism in trauma: IL-1 beta is required for the production of ciliary neurotrophic factor. *J Immunol 165*:2232-2239.

Holmin S, Mathiesen T (2000) Intracerebral administration of interleukin-1beta and induction of inflammation, apoptosis, and vasogenic edema. *J Neurosurg 92*:108-120.

Hurley SD, Olschowka JA, O'Banion MK (2002) Cyclooxygenase inhibition as a strategy to ameliorate brain injury. *J Neurotrauma 19*:1-15.

Ihn H (2002) Pathogenesis of fibrosis: role of TGF-beta and CTGF. *Curr Opin Rheumatol 14*:681-685.

Isaksson J, Farooque M, Olsson Y (2005) Improved functional outcome after spinal cord injury in iNOS-deficient mice. *Spinal Cord 43*:167-170.

Jafarian-Tehrani M, Louin G, Royo NC, Besson VC, Bohme GA, Plotkine M, Marchand-Verrecchia C (2005) 1400W, a potent selective inducible NOS inhibitor, improves histopathological outcome following traumatic brain injury in rats. *Nitric Oxide 12*:61-69.

John GR, Lee SC, Brosnan CF (2003) Cytokines: powerful regulators of glial cell activation. *Neuroscientist 9*:10-22.

Jones NC, Constantin D, Gibson CL, Prior MJ, Morris PG, Marsden CA, Murphy S (2004) A detrimental role for nitric oxide synthase-2 in the pathology resulting from acute cerebral injury. *J Neuropathol Exp Neurol 63*:708-720.

Kim GM, Xu J, Song SK, Yan P, Ku G, Xu XM, Hsu CY (2001) Tumor necrosis factor receptor deletion reduces nuclear factor-kappaB activation, cellular inhibitor of apoptosis protein 2 expression, and functional recovery after traumatic spinal cord injury. *J Neurosci 21*:6617-6625.

Kinoshita K, Chatzipanteli K, Vitarbo E, Truettner JS, Alonso OF, Dietrich WD (2002) Interleukin-1beta messenger ribonucleic acid and protein levels after fluid-percussion brain injury in rats: importance of injury severity and brain temperature. *Neurosurgery 51*:195-203; discussion 203.

Kita T, Tanaka T, Tanaka N, Kinoshita Y (2000) The role of tumor necrosis factor-alpha in diffuse axonal injury following fluid-percussive brain injury in rats. *Int J Legal Med 113*:221-228.

Knoblach SM, Faden AI (2000) Cortical interleukin-1 beta elevation after traumatic brain injury in the rat: no effect of two selective antagonists on motor recovery. *Neurosci Lett 289*:5-8.

Kunz T, Marklund N, Hillered L, Oliw EH (2002) Cyclooxygenase-2, prostaglandin synthases, and prostaglandin H2 metabolism in traumatic brain injury in the rat. *J Neurotrauma 19*:1051-1064.

Kwak EK, Kim JW, Kang KS, Lee YH, Hua QH, Park TI, Park JY, Sohn YK (2005) The role of inducible nitric oxide synthase following spinal cord injury in rat. *J Korean Med Sci 20*:663-669.

Kyrkanides S, O'Banion MK, Whiteley PE, Daeschner JC, Olschowka JA (2001) Enhanced glial activation and expression of specific CNS inflammation-related molecules in aged versus young rats following cortical stab injury. *J Neuroimmunol 119*:269-277.

La Rosa G, Cardali S, Genovese T, Conti A, Di Paola R, La Torre D, Cacciola F, Cuzzocrea S (2004) Inhibition of the nuclear factor-kappaB activation with pyrrolidine dithiocarbamate attenuating inflammation and oxidative stress after experimental spinal cord trauma in rats. *J Neurosurg Spine 1*:311-321.

Lacroix S, Chang L, Rose-John S, Tuszynski MH (2002) Delivery of hyper-interleukin-6 to the injured spinal cord increases neutrophil and macrophage infiltration and inhibits axonal growth. *J Comp Neurol 454*:213-228.

Lagord C, Berry M, Logan A (2002) Expression of TGFbeta2 but not TGFbeta1 correlates with the deposition of scar tissue in the lesioned spinal cord. *Mol Cell Neurosci 20*:69-92.

Lee YL, Shih K, Bao P, Ghirnikar RS, Eng LF (2000) Cytokine chemokine expression in contused rat spinal cord. *Neurochem Int 36*:417-425.

Logan A, Berry M, Gonzalez AM, Frautschy SA, Sporn MB, Baird A (1994) Effects of transforming growth factor beta 1 on scar production in the injured central nervous system of the rat. *Eur J Neurosci 6*:355-363.

Lotocki G, Alonso OF, Dietrich WD, Keane RW (2004) Tumor necrosis factor receptor 1 and its signaling intermediates are recruited to lipid rafts in the traumatized brain. *J Neurosci 24*:11010-11016.

Ma M, Wei P, Wei T, Ransohoff RM, Jakeman LB (2004) Enhanced axonal growth into a spinal cord contusion injury site in a strain of mouse (129X1/SvJ) with a diminished inflammatory response. *J Comp Neurol 474*:469-486.

Marriott DR, Wilkin GP, Wood JN (1991) Substance P-induced release of prostaglandins from astrocytes: regional specialisation and correlation with phosphoinositol metabolism. *J Neurochem 56*:259-265.

Minghetti L, Levi G (1998) Microglia as effector cells in brain damage and repair: focus on prostanoids and nitric oxide. *Prog Neurobiol 54*:99-125.

Moon LD, Fawcett JW (2001) Reduction in CNS scar formation without concomitant increase in axon regeneration following treatment of adult rat brain with a combination of antibodies to TGFbeta1 and beta2. *Eur J Neurosci 14*:1667-1677.

Moore AH, Olschowka JA, O'Banion MK (2004) Intraparenchymal administration of interleukin-1beta induces cyclooxygenase-2-mediated expression of membrane- and cytosolic-associated prostaglandin E synthases in mouse brain. *J Neuroimmunol 148*:32-40.

Morganti-Kossmann MC, Rancan M, Stahel PF, Kossmann T (2002) Inflammatory response in acute traumatic brain injury: a double-edged sword. *Curr Opin Crit Care 8*:101-105.

Mueller CA, Schluesener HJ, Conrad S, Meyermann R, Schwab JM (2003a) Spinal cord injury induces lesional expression of the proinflammatory and antiangiogenic cytokine EMAP II. *J Neurotrauma 20*:1007-1015.

Mueller CA, Schluesener HJ, Conrad S, Meyermann R, Schwab JM (2003b) Lesional expression of a proinflammatory and antiangiogenic cytokine EMAP II confined to endothelium and microglia/macrophages during secondary damage following experimental traumatic brain injury. *J Neuroimmunol 135*:1-9.

Nesic O, Xu GY, McAdoo D, High KW, Hulsebosch C, Perez-Pol R (2001) IL-1 receptor antagonist prevents apoptosis and caspase-3 activation after spinal cord injury. *J Neurotrauma 18*:947-956.

Nomoto Y, Yamamoto M, Fukushima T, Kimura H, Ohshima K, Tomonaga M (2001) Expression of nuclear factor kappaB and tumor necrosis factor alpha in the mouse brain after experimental thermal ablation injury. *Neurosurgery 48*:158-166.

Nonaka M, Chen XH, Pierce JE, Leoni MJ, McIntosh TK, Wolf JA, Smith DH (1999) Prolonged activation of NF-kappaB following traumatic brain injury in rats. *J Neurotrauma 16*:1023-1034.

Okada S, Nakamura M, Mikami Y, Shimazaki T, Mihara M, Ohsugi Y, Iwamoto Y, Yoshizaki K, Kishimoto T, Toyama Y, Okano H (2004) Blockade of interleukin-6 receptor suppresses reactive astrogliosis and ameliorates functional recovery in experimental spinal cord injury. *J Neurosci Res 76*:265-276.

Otto VI, Stahel PF, Rancan M, Kariya K, Shohami E, Yatsiv I, Eugster HP, Kossmann T, Trentz O, Morganti-Kossmann MC (2001) Regulation of chemokines and chemokine receptors after experimental closed head injury. *Neuroreport 12*:2059-2064.

Pan JZ, Ni L, Sodhi A, Aguanno A, Young W, Hart RP (2002) Cytokine activity contributes to induction of inflammatory cytokine mRNAs in spinal cord following contusion. *J Neurosci Res 68*:315-322.

Pearse DD, Chatzipanteli K, Marcillo AE, Bunge MB, Dietrich WD (2003) Comparison of iNOS inhibition by antisense and pharmacological inhibitors after spinal cord injury. *J Neuropathol Exp Neurol 62*:1096-1107.

Penkowa M, Moos T, Carrasco J, Hadberg H, Molinero A, Bluethmann H, Hidalgo J (1999) Strongly compromised inflammatory response to brain injury in interleukin-6-deficient mice. *Glia 25*:343-357.

Perrin FE, Lacroix S, Aviles-Trigueros M, David S (2005) Involvement of monocyte chemoattractant protein-1, macrophage inflammatory protein-1alpha and interleukin-1beta in Wallerian degeneration. *Brain 128*:854-866.

Popovich PG, Wei P, Stokes BT (1997) Cellular inflammatory response after spinal cord injury in Sprague-Dawley and Lewis rats. *J Comp Neurol 377*:443-464.

Qiu J, Whalen MJ, Lowenstein P, Fiskum G, Fahy B, Darwish R, Aarabi B, Yuan J, Moskowitz MA (2002) Upregulation of the Fas receptor death-inducing signaling complex after traumatic brain injury in mice and humans. *J Neurosci 22*:3504-3511.

Ransohoff RM, Hamilton TA, Tani M, Stoler MH, Shick HE, Major JA, Estes ML, Thomas DM, Tuohy VK (1993) Astrocyte expression of mRNA encoding cytokines IP-10 and JE/MCP-1 in experimental autoimmune encephalomyelitis. *FASEB J 7*:592-600.

Rappert A, Bechmann I, Pivneva T, Mahlo J, Biber K, Nolte C, Kovac AD, Gerard C, Boddeke HW, Nitsch R, Kettenmann H (2004) CXCR3-dependent microglial recruitment is essential for dendrite loss after brain lesion. *J Neurosci 24*:8500-8509.

Ravikumar R, Flora G, Geddes JW, Hennig B, Toborek M (2004) Nicotine attenuates oxidative stress, activation of redox-regulated transcription factors and induction of proinflammatory genes in compressive spinal cord trauma. *Brain Res Mol Brain Res 124*:188-198.

Resnick DK, Graham SH, Dixon CE, Marion DW (1998) Role of cyclooxygenase 2 in acute spinal cord injury. *J Neurotrauma 15*:1005-1013.

Roof RL, Hall ED (2000) Estrogen-related gender difference in survival rate and cortical blood flow after impact-acceleration head injury in rats. *J Neurotrauma 17*:1155-1169.

Rostworowski M, Balasingam V, Chabot S, Owens T, Yong VW (1997) Astrogliosis in the neonatal and adult murine brain post-trauma: elevation of inflammatory cytokines and the lack of requirement for endogenous interferon-gamma. *J Neurosci 17*:3664-3674.

Saas P, Boucraut J, Quiquerez AL, Schnuriger V, Perrin G, Desplat-Jego S, Bernard D, Walker PR, Dietrich PY (1999) CD95 (Fas/Apo-1) as a receptor governing astrocyte apoptotic or inflammatory responses: a key role in brain inflammation? *J Immunol 162*:2326-2333.

Sanz O, Acarin L, Gonzalez B, Castellano B (2002) NF-kappaB and IkappaBalpha expression following traumatic brain injury to the immature rat brain. *J Neurosci Res 67*:772-780.

Schluesener HJ, Seid K, Zhao Y, Meyermann R (1997) Localization of endothelial-monocyte-activating polypeptide II (EMAP II), a novel proinflammatory cytokine, to lesions of experimental autoimmune encephalomyelitis, neuritis and uveitis: expression by monocytes and activated microglial cells. *Glia 20*:365-372.

Schnell L, Fearn S, Klassen H, Schwab ME, Perry VH (1999) Acute inflammatory responses to mechanical lesions in the CNS: differences between brain and spinal cord. *Eur J Neurosci 11*:3648-3658.

Seibert K, Zhang Y, Leahy K, Hauser S, Masferrer J, Perkins W, Lee L, Isakson P (1994) Pharmacological and biochemical demonstration of the role of cyclooxygenase 2 in inflammation and pain. *Proc Natl Acad Sci U S A 91*:12013-12017.

Sharma HS, Winkler T, Stalberg E, Gordh T, Alm P, Westman J (2003) Topical application of TNF-alpha antiserum attenuates spinal cord trauma induced edema formation, microvascular permeability disturbances and cell injury in the rat. *Acta Neurochir Suppl 86*:407-413.

Sinz EH, Kochanek PM, Dixon CE, Clark RS, Carcillo JA, Schiding JK, Chen M, Wisniewski SR, Carlos TM, Williams D, DeKosky ST, Watkins SC, Marion DW, Billiar TR (1999) Inducible nitric oxide synthase is an endogenous neuroprotectant after traumatic brain injury in rats and mice. *J Clin Invest 104*:647-656.

Sroga JM, Jones TB, Kigerl KA, McGaughy VM, Popovich PG (2003) Rats and mice exhibit distinct inflammatory reactions after spinal cord injury. *J Comp Neurol 462*:223-240.

Strauss KI, Barbe MF, Marshall RM, Raghupathi R, Mehta S, Narayan RK (2000) Prolonged cyclooxygenase-2 induction in neurons and glia following traumatic brain injury in the rat. *J Neurotrauma 17*:695-711.

Streit WJ, Semple-Rowland SL, Hurley SD, Miller RC, Popovich PG, Stokes BT (1998) Cytokine mRNA profiles in contused spinal cord and axotomized facial nucleus suggest a beneficial role for inflammation and gliosis. *Exp Neurol 152*:74-87.

Sugiura S, Lahav R, Han J, Kou SY, Banner LR, de Pablo F, Patterson PH (2000) Leukaemia inhibitory factor is required for normal inflammatory responses to injury in the peripheral and central nervous systems in vivo and is chemotactic for macrophages in vitro. *Eur J Neurosci 12*:457-466.

Tehranian R, Andell-Jonsson S, Beni SM, Yatsiv I, Shohami E, Bartfai T, Lundkvist J, Iverfeldt K (2002) Improved recovery and delayed cytokine induction after closed head injury in mice with central overexpression of the secreted isoform of the interleukin-1 receptor antagonist. *J Neurotrauma 19*:939-951.

Tonai T, Taketani Y, Ueda N, Nishisho T, Ohmoto Y, Sakata Y, Muraguchi M, Wada K, Yamamoto S (1999) Possible involvement of interleukin-1 in cyclooxygenase-2 induction after spinal cord injury in rats. *J Neurochem 72*:302-309.

Toulmond S, Rothwell NJ (1995) Interleukin-1 receptor antagonist inhibits neuronal damage caused by fluid percussion injury in the rat. *Brain Res 671*:261-266.

Tuna M, Polat S, Erman T, Ildan F, Gocer AI, Tuna N, Tamer L, Kaya M, Cetinalp E (2001) Effect of anti-rat interleukin-6 antibody after spinal cord injury in the rat: inducible nitric oxide synthase expression, sodium- and potassium-activated, magnesium-dependent adenosine-5'-triphosphatase and superoxide dismutase activation, and ultrastructural changes. *J Neurosurg 95*:64-73.

Vanegas H, Schaible HG (2001) Prostaglandins and cyclooxygenases [correction of cycloxygenases] in the spinal cord. *Prog Neurobiol 64*:327-363.

Wajant H, Pfizenmaier K, Scheurich P (2003) Non-apoptotic Fas signaling. *Cytokine Growth Factor Rev 14*:53-66.

Wang CX, Olschowka JA, Wrathall JR (1997) Increase of interleukin-1beta mRNA and protein in the spinal cord following experimental traumatic injury in the rat. *Brain Res 759*:190-196.

Wang XJ, Kong KM, Qi WL, Ye WL, Song PS (2005) Interleukin-1 beta induction of neuron apoptosis depends on p38 mitogen-activated protein kinase activity after spinal cord injury. *Acta Pharmacol Sin 26*:934-942.

Westergren-Thorsson G, Schmidtchen A, Sarnstrand B, Fransson LA, Malmstrom A (1992) Transforming growth factor-beta induces selective increase of proteoglycan production and changes in the copolymeric structure of dermatan sulphate in human skin fibroblasts. *Eur J Biochem 205*:277-286.

Woodroofe MN, Sarna GS, Wadhwa M, Hayes GM, Loughlin AJ, Tinker A, Cuzner ML (1991) Detection of interleukin-1 and interleukin-6 in adult rat brain, following mechanical injury, by in vivo microdialysis: evidence of a role for microglia in cytokine production. *J Neuroimmunol 33*:227-236.

Xu J, Fan G, Chen S, Wu Y, Xu XM, Hsu CY (1998) Methylprednisolone inhibition of TNF-alpha expression and NF-kB activation after spinal cord injury in rats. *Brain Res Mol Brain Res 59*:135-142.

Yan P, Li Q, Kim GM, Xu J, Hsu CY, Xu XM (2001) Cellular localization of tumor necrosis factor-alpha following acute spinal cord injury in adult rats. *J Neurotrauma 18*:563-568.

Yan P, Xu J, Li Q, Chen S, Kim GM, Hsu CY, Xu XM (1999) Glucocorticoid receptor expression in the spinal cord after traumatic injury in adult rats. *J Neurosci 19*:9355-9363.

Yang K, Mu XS, Hayes RL (1995) Increased cortical nuclear factor-kappa B (NF-kappa B) DNA binding activity after traumatic brain injury in rats. *Neurosci Lett 197*:101-104.

Yang L, Jones NR, Blumbergs PC, Van Den Heuvel C, Moore EJ, Manavis J, Sarvestani GT, Ghabriel MN (2005) Severity-dependent expression of pro-inflammatory cytokines in traumatic spinal cord injury in the rat. *J Clin Neurosci 12*:276-284.

Yune TY, Lee SM, Kim SJ, Park HK, Oh YJ, Kim YC, Markelonis GJ, Oh TH (2004) Manganese superoxide dismutase induced by TNF-beta is regulated transcriptionally by NF-kappaB after spinal cord injury in rats. *J Neurotrauma 21*:1778-1794.

Zurita M, Vaquero J, Zurita I (2001) Presence and significance of CD-95 (Fas/APO1) expression after spinal cord injury. *J Neurosurg 94*:257-264.

In: Inflammation Research Perspectives
Editor: Giacomo T. Romano, pp. 81-112 ISBN: 978-1-60021-845-3

Chapter V

INFLAMMATION AND THE ROLE OF IMMUNE MEDIATORS IN THE PATHOPHYSIOLOGY OF ISCHEMIC STROKE

Christoph Kleinschnitz and Guido Stoll
Department of Neurology, Julius-Maximilians Universität, Wuerzburg, Germany

ABSTRACT

This chapter summerizes the complex interactions of immune cells and mediators in developing ischemic brain lesions and reviews current concepts on their role in neurotoxicity and –protection.

Inflammation has so far mainly been studied in the context of autoimmunity and infections of the nervous system. Only recently it has been recognized that inflammatory responses which involve hematogenous leukocytes, local microglia and immune mediators exert important functions in the pathophysiology of cerebral ischemia, a primarily non-immune lesion paradigm. Cerebral ischemia leads to immediate activation of microglia and to a temporarily graded infiltration of granulocytes, T-cells, and finally macrophages. Early microglial activation is accompanied by the upregulation of cytokines in ischemic brain lesions, and cellular adhesion molecules on corresponding endothelial cells within hours. Attenuation of microglial responses and blocking of immune mediators ameliorate ischemic brain injury in some settings suggesting a detrimental role in infarct development. Tumor necrosis factor (TNF)-alpha, members of the interleukin (IL)-1 family, and nitric oxide have been identified as main players in delayed neuronal cell death. In contrast to granulocytes and lymphocytes, macrophage entry into ischemic lesions appears to be delayed as revealed in vivo by iron contrast-enhanced magnetic resonance imaging (MRI). Thus, macrophages play a major role in tissue remodelling rather than injury.

Surprisingly, inflammation also confers neuroprotection in the brain. After hypoxic or chemical preconditioning rendering neurons less susceptible to subsequent hypoxemia, neuroprotective effects are mediated by cytokines and hematopoietic growth factors. Similarly manipulating the immune system by oral or nasal toleralization against myelin and cell adhesion proteins protects against ischemic brain injury. These beneficial effects are transferable to naive animals by T-cells.

1. INTRODUCTION: PATHOPHYSIOLOGY AND ANIMAL MODELS OF CEREBRAL ISCHEMIA

Ischemic stroke has challenged the position of cardiovascular disorders and represents the second leading cause of death among industrialized nations. The cellular pathomechanisms involved in ischemic brain damage are still incompletely understood and despite intense research activity, only one therapeutic treatment option, fibrinolysis, has been approved by the FDA until today. During the last ten years the concepts on the mechanisms of secondary infarct growth have substantially changed, now involving inflammatory and immunological responses. This chapter summarizes recent insights into the role of inflammatory mediators such as chemokines and cytokines, and immune cells in stroke development. In the following a short description introduces basic pathophysiological events at the early stages of ischemic neuronal cells death which culminates into a robust secondary inflammatory response. We will also briefly describe rodent models of cerebral ischemia commonly used in experimental stroke research.

After focal cessation of cerebral blood flow the delivery of oxygen, glucose and other substrates is restricted within the brain region supplied by the occluded artery. As an early consequence of ischemia membrane-bound transporters, which depend on permanent energy supply, are disturbed and the maintenance of ionic gradients fails. This leads to further depolarization of neurons, subsequent release of excitatory amino acids (glutamate) and finally dramatic Ca2+ influx (Dirnagl et al., 1999). Ca2+ serves as an universal second messenger activating proteolytic enzymes, facilitating free-radical formation and release of glutamate, mediators that maintain a circulus vitiosus.

There is increasing evidence that the time period during which brain infarctions develop and grow lasts longer than previously believed. In the centre of the ischemic territory where cerebral blood flow is most severly reduced, irreversible necrotic tissue damage involving endthelial, neuronal and glial cells occurs within minutes. Contrastingly, in the surrounding periphery (so-called penumbra), where blood flow is decreased but reaches a certain threshold to keep structural integrity, neurons remain viable for a prolonged period (Garcia et al., 1993; Furlan et al., 1996; Marchal et al., 1996). Depending on the extent of collateral artery supply or reperfusion of the occluded artery the infarcts further grow into the penumbra zone either by necrotic cell death or by delayed neuronal cell death (apoptosis), a process that requires sustained biosynthesis of enzymes (caspases) that lead to self-destruction of neurons. As outlined below, generation of inflammatory mediators (e. g. tumor necrosis factor (TNF), interleukin (IL)-1, inducible nitric oxide synthase (iNOS), cyclooxygenase (COX)-2) by activated microglia and infiltrating macrophages as well as the production of oxygen- and nitrogen-based free radicals have been invoked in this process.

For the study of the underlying pathomechanisms of ischemic brain lesions, several animal models have been developed which differ with respect to surgical techniques, infarct size and reproducibility (Ginsberg and Busto, 1989). Most frequently, surgical occlusion of major brain arteries is applied in rodents. Permanent occlusion of the middle cerebral artery (MACO) at proximal sites, e. g. by an intraluminal thread, causes total infarctions of the neocortex and basal ganglia. In this model subsequent infarct growth has been observed between six and 72 hrs. In human stroke initial vessel occlusion, e. g. via embolic thrombi is often followed by arterial reperfusion. This situation can be mimicked in the MCAO paradigm by withdrawing of the intraluminal thread (transient MCAO) which significantly modifies stroke development (Memezawa et al., 1992; Zhang et al., 1997). Ischemic periods below 30 minutes lead to restricted infarctions in the caudatoputamen and only partly affect the neocortex because ischemic tissue is salvaged by reperfusion. If reperfusion is further delayed, neocortical infarctions will increase since the surrounding penumbra, where cerebral blood flow is critically reduced, is subsequently involved into the definite infarct area.

One major disadvantage of the above mentioned MACO models is variability of the initial infarct localization and size. This is due to differences concerning surgical procedures and thread size, strain dependencies and interindividual alterations of vascular collaterals (Ginsberg and Busto 1989; Maeda et al., 1998; Gerriets et al., 2004). Therefore, specific regions of interest, such as the necrotic infarct core, the peripheral border zone with delayed neuronal death and the non-ischemic contralateral cortex, are difficult to differentiate in the MCAO models. As an alternative model photochemically-induced cortical infarction (photothrombosis, PT) ensures high reproducibility of infarct size and clear delineation of the infarct boundaries (Watson et al., 1985; Schroeter et al., 2001a). After systemic injection of the photosensitive dye rose bengal the brain is focally illuminated through the intact skull. This leads to free radical formation, endothelial damage and platelet aggregation, which is supposed to induce thrombotic occlusion of small cerebral vessels leading to cone-shaped cortical infarctions. However, recent studies have questioned the paradigma that the development of photothrombotic lesions depends on platelet- or plasmatic coagulation-derived thrombus formation (Frederix et al., 2007; Kleinschnitz et al., in press). Functional blockade or complete depletion of platelets or the plasmatic coagulation did not alter infarct size after cortical PT indicating that other pathophysiological mechanisms, e. g. edema formation or inflammation must be involved in photothrombotic tissue damage. These unexpected findings reveal differences in mechanisms of tissue injury induced by PT as compared to focal ischemia induced by MCAO, where platelet activation and the intrinsic coagulation pathway are instrumental (Kleinschnitz et al., 2006; 2007). As a consequence, the PT model should not be used to mimick ischemic brain infarctions but might serve as useful tool to study lesion-associated blood-brain-barrier alterations and secondary inflammatory mechanisms.

2. The Cellular Inflammatory Response to Cerebral Ischemia: Basic Observations

2.1. Granulocytes

Granulocytes are the predominant cell type that massively infiltrate ischemic brain areas during the early phase of transient or permanent cerebral ischemia (Kochanek and

Hallenbeck, 1992). These hematogenous cells accumulate in cerebral vessels within hours and subsequently invade the infarct core and its boundary zone. This process peaks after 24 hrs while the number of granulocytes rapidly declines thereafter (Garcia et al., 1994). Within the second week after infarction most of the granulocytes have disappeared.

Leukocyte recruitment into ischemic brain tissue is caused by the up-regulation of cell adhesion molecules on hypoxic endothelial cells and of chemokines that are released from the site of injury to attract hematogenous cells. As a first step the velocity of leukocytes in the blood stream is focally reduced as they loosely attach to endothelial cells via selectins (E-selectin, P-selectin, L-selectin). Then, firm adhesion of leukocytes to the endothelium is mediated by integrin interactions. While leukocytes constitutively express the ligands (LFA-1, VLA-4, CD11b/CD18) on their surface the corresponding counterreceptors such as ICAM-1 (intercellular adhesion molecule-1) and VCAM-1 (vascular cell adhesion molecule-1) on the endothelial cells require specific induction and thereby determine the location of leukocyte/endothelial cell interaction. After cerebral ischemia ICAM-1 was shown to be expressed as early as 3 hrs in intraparenchymal blood vessels of the ischemic cortex (Jander et al., 1995; Zhang et al., 1995a). Maximum ICAM-1 levels were reached between 6 and 12 hrs and expression persisted for several days. Other members of the cell adhesion family, e. g. VCAM-1 and ELAM-1 (endothelial leukocyte adhesion molecule-1) were likewise upregulated in focal cerebral ischemia and showed a temporal expression profile similiar to ICAM-1 (Wang et al., 1995a; Jander et al., 1996; Del Zoppo et al., 2000).

Functionally, there is evidence that intravascular granulocyte accumulation reduces blood flow in the reperfusion period and thereby contributes to extension of infarctions in transient cerebral ischemia (no-reflow phenomenon). Infarct volume and the number of apoptotic cells and invading granulocytes were reduced by treatment with antibodies directed against the CD11/CD18 complex present on granulocytes of rats subjected to transient MCAO (Chopp et al., 1996). In line with these results, blocking of the corresponding ligand on endothelial cells, ICAM-1, strongly reduced stroke volumes at day 2 by 80 % (Zhang et al., 1995b) and ICAM-1 knock out mice displayed a fivefold decrease in infarct size (Conolly et al., 1996). However, systemic application of anti-leukocyte antibodies in permanent MCAO was not effective (Zhang et al., 1995b). This is most likely due to the fact that infiltrating granulocytes adhere to the microvasculature via the ICAM-1/CD11 pathway and mechanically disconnect dependent parenchyma from reperfusion. Prolonged hypoxia then leads to extension of the infarct area into the penumbra zone. In a recent human stroke trial, however, monoclonal anti-ICAM-1 antibody (enlimomab) failed and case fatality rate was significantly higher in the enlimomab patient group (EAST, 2001). These adverse events of enlimomab were most likely due to the unexpected activation of neutrophil granulocytes, complement and endothelial cells (Vuorte et al., 1999). As another prospective clinical approach subcutaneous injections of interferon-beta (IFN-β) which has multiple immunomodulatory effects including down-regulation of cell adhesion molecules, significantly reduced lesion volumes after experimental cerebral ischemia. This therapeutic effect still persisted when the substance was applied delayed 6 hrs after stroke onset (Veldhuis et al., 2003). IFN- β treated animals showed preservation of blood-brain barrier integrity and reduced neutrophil and monocyte infiltration into the ischemic tissue.

2.2. T Cells

T cells usually infiltrate the CNS during infectious or autoimmune disorders such as experimental autoimmune encephalomyelitis (EAE) and human multiple sclerosis (MS) where they serve as inducer cells of antigen-specific immune responses (Wekerle et al., 1986; Stoll et al., 1993). Numerous CD5+ T cells have also been detected in ischemic brain lesions after permanent MCAO and PT which was surprising (Schroeter et al., 1994; Jander et al., 1995). These cells started to infiltrate the infarct region from day 1 onwards. At day 3 their number had increased and reached a peak at later time points around day 7. T cells were preferentially located in the boundary zone of the infarctions in close vicinity to blood vessels (Becker et al., 1997; Stoll et al., 1998).

Several recent studies could elegantly demonstrate that the role of T cells is not restricted to the late reperfusion phase but rather, these cells have been strongly implicated also in the early stage of infarct development. 24 hours after 60 min middle cerebral artery occlusion brain infarct volumes were significantly reduced in mice deficient in lymphocytes (RAG1 KO mice) (Yilmaz et al., 2006; Kleinschnitz and Stoll, unpublished observations). Subtype analysis revealed that CD8+ T cells, and to a lesser extent CD4+ T cells, are important in the development of postischemic cerebral infarcts, while B cell deficiency did not alter infarct volumes following tMCAO (Yilamaz et al., 2006). Similar results were obtained in severe combined immunodeficent (SCID) mice lacking both, T and B cells (Hurn et al., 2007). The mechanism by which T cell deficiency mediates neuroprotection in experimental stroke seems to be at least partly mediated by reduced interactions between lymphocytes and platelets in the cerebral microcvasculature leading to improved tissue reperfusion. RAG1 KO mice displayed lower numbers of adherent leukocytes and platelets in cerebral venules after tMCAO (Yilmaz et al., 2006). In line with these observations mice lacking the membrane glycoprotein CD40 or its receptor CD40 ligand (CD40L), which are both expressed on various cell types including T cells, platelets or endothelial cells and play a key role in inflammation, e. g. through the induction of cellular adhesion molecules and the recruitment of immune cells (Xu and Song, 2004), were highly protected from experimental cerebral ischemia (Ishikawa et al., 2005). In addition, mice with null mutations of lymphocyte function-associated antigen-1 (LFA-1) or macrophage-1 (MAC-1), which are both critically involved in leukocyte/platelet interactions, exhibited significant reductions in infarct volume at day 1 after tMCAO (Arumugam et al., 2004). Again, the amount of T cells and platelets binding to the ischemic endothelium was highly diminished compared to WT controls.

In contrast to primarily inflammatory diseases the time period between the ischemic lesion and T cell infiltration is too short for the generation of systemic, antigen-specific signaling. Thus, T cell recruitment and T cell effector funtions are likely to be antigen non-specific in cerebral ischemia. The specific signal that attracts T cells and keeps them in the CNS parenchyma is unknown at present although it is likely that up-regulation of cell adhesion molecules is involved in this process. The functional relevance of the T cell response in cerebral ischemia is not fully understood yet but might also be connected to neuroprotection and immune tolerance (see also section 4.) or the contribution of regulatory T cells at later stages after focal cerebral ischemia (Offner et al., 2006).

2.3. Macrophages and Microglia

As a third group of inflammatory cells, monocytes enter the brain after focal cerebral ischemia and transform into phagocytes (Garcia et al., 1994; Jander et al., 1995). The pool of phagocytes in cerebral ischemia, however, also involves microglia, the resident „macrophages“ of the brain. Microglia are locally activated after ischemia, loose their ramified appearance in the normal brain, and thereby become indistinguishable from blood-borne macrophages on morphological grounds. Moreover, most immunocytochemical markers used to differentiate between cell types are shared between macrophages and microglia, making the differentiation an intrinsic problem (Flaris et al., 1993). After permanent MCAO phagocytes were located in the brain parenchyma within 12 hrs and further increased in number up to day 14 (Schroeter et al., 1994; Rupalla et al., 1998). As early as 3 days after MCAO the entire infarct area was covered by phagocytes (Schroeter et al., 1994) which completely cleared cell debris within the next four weeks. In the PT model of focal cerebral ischemia the location of phagocytes was different since they were arranged in a rim-like fashion around the ischemic core during the first week and invaded the lesion centre with a delay of several days (Jander et al., 1995). The problem of distinguishing between macrophage infiltration from the circulation and local microglial responses could recently be solved elegantly by a novel magnetic resonance imaging (MRI) technique (Figure 1 A-D). Superparamagnetic iron particles (SPIO) injected into the circulation are rapidly taken up by circulating macrophages and cleared by the reticuloendothelial system of the liver and the spleen. When macrophages are attracted to damaged tissue during nerve injury or cerebral ischemia they take with them their SPIO particles that serve as a paramagnetic contrast agent detectable on MRI (Chen et al., 1999; Bendszus and Stoll, 2003; Kleinschnitz et al., 2003). Accumulation of SPIO-laden macrophages led to signal loss on T2-weighted MR images. Using this technique we could show that hematogenous macrophages are recruited with a delay of several days to ischemic brain lesions, and that transformed microglia account for most phagocytes at early stages of infarct development (Figure 1 A-D). Interestingly, macrophage recruitment was independent from the breakdown of the blood-brain barrier (BBB), which was present immediately after ischemia and persisted for weeks, while macrophage recruitment was restricted to day 5-9 after focal ischemia in the PT model. A similar delay in macrophage recruitment was recently confirmed in a pilot study in human stroke (Saleh et al., 2004). Taken together these studies suggest that macrophages play a role in tissue remodelling and repair rather than neuronal injury because they appear at a stage in which delayed neuronal cell death has already ceased (Isenmann et al., 1998). Rather microglial activation plays a detrimental role early. Accordingly, the importance of microglia in stroke development has been substantiated pharmacologically. The tetracycline derivative minocyclin attenuated microglial responses and concurrently reduced infarct volumes (Yrjanheikki et al., 1999).

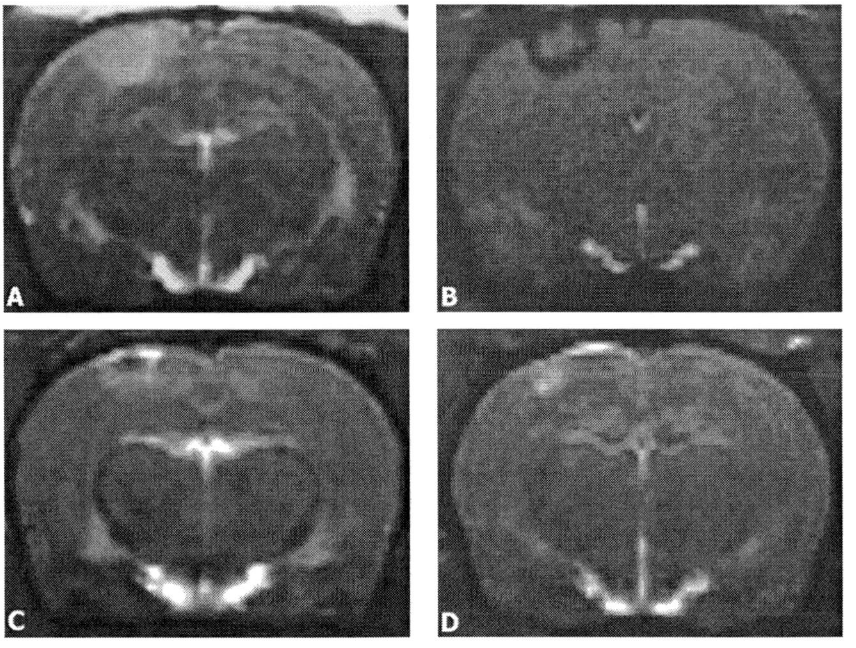

Figure 1. In-vivo assessment of active macrophage infiltration by magnetic resonance (MR) imaging as indicated by focal signal loss: Coronal CISS-weighed MR images (slice thickness 1 mm) of photothrombotic infarcts at day 3 (A), 6 (B), 8 (C) and 14 (D). Animals received superparamagnetic iron (SPIO) particles systemically always 24 hrs before MRI. Infarcts appeared as hyperintense lesions at early stages of infarct development due to tissue damage and edema formation (A). SPIO-laden macrophages are not yet present. At day 6 signal loss (black rim) indicative of local iron accumulation was apparent at the outer margins of infarcts (B), at day 8 the core of the lesions exhibited signal loss, while the periphery appeared hyperintense again (C). These black areas of signal loss on MRI represent infarct regions with recent macrophage infiltration from the circulation. At day 14 lesions were entirely hyperintense again and had shrunken due to tissue remodelling and scar formation (D). At this late time point of infarct reorganization no more macrophage infiltration takes place. Reprinted from Kleinschnitz et al. (2003) Journal of Cerebral Blood Flow & Metabolism 23:1356-1361 with permission of the publisher.

Macrophage infiltration after focal cerebral ischemia is paralleled by the expression of monocyte chemoattractant protein-1 (MCP-1) (Kim et al., 1995; Wang et al., 1995b). MCP-1 mRNA was elevated up to day 5, and MCP-1 protein was expressed by endothelial and „macrophage-like“ cells (Kim et al., 1995). Furthermore, astrocytes surrounding the ischemic tissue as well as reactive microglia are possible sources of MCP-1 (Gourmala et al., 1997) These findings suggest that both chemokines and cell adhesion molecules are involved in the coordinated recruitment of inflammatory cells to focal ischemic lesions (see also section 2.1.).

Microglia and macrophages associated with ischemic brain lesions in the rat exhibit an unusual immunophenotype. Microglia/macrophages commonly express CD4 in CNS lesion paradigms. In addition, a novel population of cells expressing the CD8 molecule was noticed in ischemic brain lesions between days 3 and 6 (Schroeter et al., 1994; Schroeter et al., 2001b; Jander et al., 1998a). At day 14 most of these cells had disappeared. The CD8 molecule is usually restricted to T cells and natural killer (NK) cells (Lawetzky et al., 1990).

However, most of the CD8+ cells in ischemic brain lesions were negative for T cell markers but expressed microglia/macrophage markers. CD8+ macrophages were exclusively located in the border zone and the core of pannecrotic brain tissue but absent in areas of selective neuronal cell death or during fibre tract degeneration. Their functional role in brain ischemia is unclear at present. In-vitro studies performed independently on alveolar macrophages showed that signalling via the CD8 molecule led to the expression of TNF, IL-1β and iNOS and stimulated the production of NO (Hirji et al., 1998). NO is regarded as a major pathogenic factor in ischemic brain damage (see also section 3.1.4.).

Although microglia is the main effector cell population of the innate immune system following CNS injuries, including cerebral ischemia (Nedergaard and Dirnagl, 2005) it still remains controversial whether activation of these cells has beneficial or detrimental effects on ischemic brain tissue (Nguyen et al., 2002; Nedergaard and Dirnagl, 2005). On the one hand, activated microglia can release proinflammatory cytokines (e. g. TNFα and IL-1β), nitric oxide and reactive oxygen species (see above), molecules, which can augment ischemic brain damage (Stoll et al., 1998; Gibson et al., 2005). In addition, attenuation of microglial activation has conferred neuroprotection in several models of neurodegeneration (Tikka et al., 2001; Kriz et al., 2002, 2003). On the other hand, increasing evidence suggests a neuroprotective role for local microglia in various CNS pathologies (Streit 2002). Exogenous application of microglia for example protects from focal and global cerebral ischemia (Neumann et al., 2006; Imai et al., 2007) and Lalancette-Hébert and co-workers could recently demonstrate that selective ablation of proliferating microglia using CD11b-thymidine kinase mutant-30 transgenic mice significantly raises brain infarct volumes after tMCAO (Lalancette-Hébert et al., 2007). This effect was probably mediated by enhanced expression of proinflammatory cytokines, increased apoptosis and less production of neurotrophic factors such as insulin-line growth factor-1 (IGF-1) although the molecular mechanisms underlying neuroprotection by microglial cells remain elusive at present.

3. The Molecular Inflammatory Response to Cerebral Ischemia: Cytokines and Nitric Oxide

3.1. Infarct and Periinfarct Regions

Cytokines serve as humoral regulators of the activation and interaction of immune cells such as T-cells, B cells and monocytes/macrophages. They thereby orchestrate immune responses in a network-like fashion (Arai et al., 1990). In the nervous system, cytokines moreover are involved in brain development and plasticity. They play a key role in the induction and effector phase of autoimmune or infectious disorders of the nervous system, in which both resident glial cells (Schwann cells, microglia, astrocytes) as well as invading leukocytes from the circulation contribute as cellular sources (Kennedy et al., 1992; Jander et al., 1998b; Merril and Jonakait, 1995). Cytokine expression is not restricted to primarily inflammatory settings, but also plays a decisive role in the pathophysiology of degenerative neurological disorders and during nerve regeneration (Mehler and Kessler; 1997; Gillen et al., 1998; Kleinschnitz et al., 2004a; Stoll et al., 2002; Stoll et al., 2004). During the last ten years the important role of cytokines in lesion development after cerebral ischemia has been recognized and the different pathways involved in exerting their neurotoxic and neuroprotective effects have been elucidated (Feuerstein et al., 1994; Stoll et al., 1998). In the following the role of three major proinflammatory cytokines IL-1, TNF, and IL-18 is discussed in detail.

3.1.1. Interleukin-1β

IL-1β is expressed at low levels in the normal brain, but is rapidly induced after cerebral ischemia. Following permanent MCAO, IL-1β mRNA significantly increases in the ischemic cortex within one hour, and reaches peak levels during the first 24 hrs. IL-1β mRNA rapidly declines thereafter (Liu et al., 1993; Buttini et al., 1994). On the protein level IL-1β is mainly expressed by ramified microglia at early stage of infarct development with an uncertain contribution of hematogenous macrophages and astrocytes later on. The specific IL-1 effects are mediated by IL-1 type I (IL-1RI) and type II (IL-RII) receptors. While IL-1RI transduces an intracellular signal, IL-1RII binds IL-1 without generating a specific signal, which means it acts as a natural IL-1 antagonist. The increase of IL-1 receptors mRNA was directly associated with the up-regulation of IL-1β (Wang et al., 1997). In addition gene expression of the physiological counteractor of IL-1β, IL-1 receptor antagonist (IL-1ra) peaks between 6 and 12 hrs after MCAO in the ischemic hemisphere and remains elevated for up to 5 days. In the healthy brain IL-1RI and IL-1RII are found on neurons of the hippocampus and on Purkinje cells of the cerebellum, while cellular expression under ischemic conditions is still unclear at present.

Pharmacological studies as well as stroke induction in genetically manipulated animals provide evidence that IL-1 is involved in ischemic brain damage (Rothwell and Luheshi, 2000). Intracerebroventricular application of IL-1β worsens brain damage after focal cerebral ischemia. It became apparent, however, that IL-1α and IL-1β have overlapping effects since single knock-out mice showed no changes in infarct size while infarct volumes in double knock-out mice lacking both the IL-1α and IL-1β gene were greatly reduced. This study and others led to the conclusion that IL-1 plays a detrimental role in infarct development (Boutin et al., 2001). IL-1 effects must be mediated by multiple receptor molecules since IL-1RI knock-out mice showed a normal response to intracerebroventricular IL-1 injections (Yamasaki et al., 1995; Stroemer et al., 1998; Touzani et al., 2002). Currently, the agonistic IL-1β effects in vivo apparently predominate over the antagonistic IL-1ra properties, although both molecules are co-induced in the infarct area. Intracerebroventricular as well as systemic injection of IL-1ra significantly reduced stroke damage (Rothwell and Luheshi, 2000; Relton et al., 1992; Garcia et al., 1995). However, it has been estimated that IL-1ra needs to be at more than 100-fold excess to fully neutralize IL-1. This is emphasized by the fact that chronic overexpression of IL-1ra in transgenic mice was not neuroprotective in a mouse model of permanent focal cerebral ischemia (Oprica et al., 2004).

Caspase-1 cleaves proIL-1 to generate biologically active IL-1β. Inhibition of caspase-1 decreased infarct volumes, which is in further support of a potentially noxious role of IL-1β in stroke (Loddick et al., 1996; Hara et al., 1997). Furthermore, mice with a mutant caspase-1 gene developed smaller infarcts, milder neurological deficits, reduced IL-1β levels and decreased DNA fragmentation after transient and permanent MCAO (Rabuffetti et al., 2000).

Besides activation of IL-1β, caspase-1 mediates apoptotic pathways and modulates the release of the proinflammatory cytokine IL-18 (see also section 3.1.3.). Thus the mitigating effects of caspase-1 elimination might not solely be due to reduction of IL-1β production. Accordingly, elevated caspase-1 gene expression in focal ischemia displayed a sustained time course in parallel to IL-18-mRNA, but did not correlate to the early and restricted expression of IL-1β mRNA (Jander et al., 2002).

3.1.2. TNF-α

As is the case with IL-1β, TNF-α is rapidly induced within the first three hours after permanent MCAO and its expression persists during the next days (Barone et al., 1997; Liu et al., 1994). A similar induction of TNF-α and IL-1β was seen in transient MCAO although baseline levels were reached earlier around day 2 (Wang et al., 1994). Unlike IL-1β, TNF-α-immunoreactivity is mainly associated with ischemic neurons in the evolving infarct and the penumbra. In addition, astrocytes, microglia, macrophages and granulocytes appear to be sources of TNF-α (Gregersen et al., 2000; Botchkina et al., 1997). In parallel with the expression of TNF-α, the corresponding TNF receptors p55 and p75 were up-regulated within six and 24 hrs, respectively. TNF receptor p55 has been implicated in transducing the cytotoxic signalling of TNF. The presence of TNF-α protein and TNF p55 receptors therefore suggests an injurious role of excessive TNF production during the acute response to cerebral ischemia (Shohami et al., 1999). Intraventricular application of TNF-α 24 hrs prior to MCAO significantly exacerbated the infarct size probably by activating capillary endothelium to a pro-adhesive state (Arvin et al., 1996). Furthermore, treatment with neutralizing antibodies or TNF-binding protein significantly reduced the cortical infarct volume (Barone et al., 1997; Shohami et al., 1999). Similar neuroprotective effects due to TNF inhibition were obtained with daxanabiolol (HU-211), a non-psychotropic cannabinoid analogue (Lecker et al., 1999) and DPH-067517, a selective inhibitor of TNF-α converting enzyme (TACE) (Wang et al., 2004). The fact that the application of TNF-α did not directly affect neurotransmitter release or free radical toxicity in cultured cerebellar granule cells allows the conclusion that TNF neurotoxicity is triggered by non-neuronal cell types. Overall, the functional role of TNF in cerebral ischemia is a double-edged sword since this cytokine can exert dose and co-factor-dependent opposing neurotoxic and neuroprotective effects (see also section 4.2.) (Shohami et al., 1999; Allen and Rothwell, 2001).

3.1.3. Interleukin-18

IL-18 belongs to the IL-1 cytokine superfamily and was originally described in a mouse model of endotoxic shock as IFN-γ inducing factor. So far, it has been the only proinflammatory cytokine which is strongly linked to the late inflammatory response in focal cerebral ischemia. In experimental stroke, IL-18 mRNA and protein expression displayed a delayed kinetics of induction starting at 24 to 48 hrs and peaking 6 days after the initial insult (Jander et al., 2002). Macrophages within the ischemic core as well as perilesional microglia were found to be the cellular source of IL-18 protein.

The expression pattern of IL-18 differs from IL-1, which is induced during the acute phase of brain ischemia showing maximum levels already within the first 4 hrs. Both cytokines are synthesized as inactive precursors requiring enzymatic cleavage by caspase-1 for conversion into fully bioactive molecules. Interestingly, the induction of caspase-1 transcripts only paralleled those of IL-18, but was not related to the time course of IL-1 expression. Furthermore, elevated IL-18 mRNA levels in ischemic brain lesions were not connected to an increase of IFN-γ mRNA, which suggests that IL-18 acts independent from IFN-γ in cerebral ischemia (Jander et al., 2002). After hypoxic brain injury in 7 days old, IL-18 deficient rats, infarct volumes were significantly reduced, which is indicative for a detrimental role of IL-18 in stroke development (Hedtjarn et al., 2002). In human stroke patients, increased IL-18 serum levels were found within 24 hrs, which were positively correlated with functional stroke scores and infarct areas on brain CT (Zaremba et al., 2003). However, compared to wild type animals, transient MCAO in IL-18 knock out mice did not cause any differences in infarct volumes after one day (Wheeler et al., 2003; Braeuninger, Kleinschnitz and Stoll, unpublished observations).

3.1.4. Interferon Regulatory Factor 1 and Nitric Oxide

Interferon regulatory factor 1 (IRF) is a transcription factor that can be activated by the proinflammatory cytokines TNF-α and IL-1β. IRF induces gene transcription of the proinflammatory cytokine IFN-γ, inducible nitric oxide synthase (iNOS) and caspase-1 (Bhat et al., 1996). At 12 hrs after focal ischemia, IRF mRNA expression was significantly up-regulated and reached its peak at day 4. One day after transient MCAO, IRF-1 immunoreactivity was observed in intravascular neutrophils that infiltrate the ischemic tissue, and in neurons at the outer border of the ischemic territory. Besides, IRF-1 immunoreactiviy was found in neurons and inflammatory cells in the brain of patients who had died 1-2 days after ischemic stroke (Alexander et al., 2003). Mice lacking the IRF gene were protected from ischemic brain damage and developed smaller infarctions and less neurological deficits (Iadecola et al., 1999). This phenomenon may be explained by the lack of nitric oxide (NO) induction although the precise molecular mechanisms underlying neuroprotection in IRF-1 knock-out mice after ischemia must further be elucidated.

NO is a small gaseous molecule with pleiotropic properties and is synthesized by the oxidation of L-arginine to L-citrulline. This reaction is catalyzed by the enzyme NO synthase (NOS), which exists in three isoforms: neuronal NOS (nNOS), endothelial NOS (eNOS) and inducible NOS (iNOS). At every stage of cerebral ischemia, an increased NO production has been observed (Iadecola, 1997a). NO can exert both protective and deleterious effects depending on the NOS isoforms and the cell types by which NO is produced. Moreover the net effects of NO are dependent on the stage of infarct development.

nNOS actitvity increased 10 min after focal ischemia and returned to normal after 60 min (Kader et al., 1993). In parallel, neurons displayed an up-regulation of nNOS mRNA and an increase in nNOS immunoreactivity (Zhang and Iadecola, 1994; Iadecola et al., 1995a; De Alba et al., 1999). Overall, nNOS activation after brain ischemia seems to be detrimental since experimental stroke studies using selective nNOS inhibitors displayed reduced infarct volumes and mice lacking nNOS were more resistant to ischemic damage after transient or permanent MCAO (Yoshida et al., 1994; Goyagi et al., 2001; Ferriero et al., 1996; Huang et al., 1994).

eNOS activity and immunoreactivity are also up-regulated after cerebral ischemia, but eNOS expression starts earlier than that of nNOS (Zhang and Iadecola, 1993; Matsuoka et al.,

1997). This isoform is predominantly found in pre- and postcapillary microvessels and is important for maintaining adequate tissue perfusion (Huang et al., 1994; Veltkamp et al., 2002). When administered within 30 min after the onset of ischemia, the NO precursor L-arginine reduces infarct size by improving blood flow in the penumbra area (Zhang and Iadecola, 1994; Morikawa et al., 1994; Dalkara et al., 1994). However, the protective effect is lost if L-arginine is administered at a time point later than 30 min after the beginning of ischemia. These findings suggest that the increase of NO production at the vascular level is protective only during early times after ischemia. In line with this hypothesis, eNOS-transgenic knock-out mice are more vulnerable to ischemic damage an effect associated with a reduced cerebral blood flow in the ischemic penumbra (Huang et al., 1996).

The third NOS isoform, iNOS, continuously induces synthesis of large amounts of NO for relatively long time periods. NO then reacts with superoxide to form peroxynitrite, a highly cytotoxic agent (Knowles and Moncada, 1994). It has been demonstrated that iNOS mRNA, protein and enzymatic activity are induced in the brain after transient or permanent ischemia in rodents (Iadecola et al., 1995a; Grandati et al., 1997) as well as in in vitro models of ischemic brain damage (Moro et al., 1998; De Alba et al., 1999; Cardenas et al., 1998). In vivo, iNOS expression began between six to twelve hrs, peaked at 96 hrs and subsided after seven days (Iadecola et al., 1997b). iNOS protein was immunohistochemically located in polymorphonuclear neutrophils, astrocytes and in vascular cells of the injured brain (Iadecola et al., 1995a; Endoh et al., 1994; Wallace and Bisland, 1994; Iadecola et al., 1996). In addition, neurons can also express iNOS under ischemic conditions (Moro et al., 1998). Similarly to nNOS, selective iNOS inhibitors have been used to explore the role of this NOS isoform in experimental stroke. When administered between 12 and 24 hrs after MCAO, these substances reduced infarct volumes by 30-40 %, which was also associated with an improvement of the observed neurological deficits (Iadecola et al., 1995b; Parmentier et al., 1999). The use of iNOS knock-out animals further confirmed the results obtained by pharmacological interventions. Transgenic iNOS null mice showed smaller infarcts and better neurological outcome than their wild type littermates (Iadecola et al., 1997b), however a resent study could not confirm these results (Prüss et al., 2007). Reduction in cerebral blood flow after MCAO did not differ between iNOS knock-out and control animals indicating that iNOS deletion had no influence on early cerebrovascular parameters. Although iNOS has been mainly implicated in brain damage based on the studies described above, a protective role in focal cerebral ischemia has also been described. The neuroprotective effect of volatile anesthetics after permanent MCAO in rats was accompanied by an induction of iNOS protein which began to increase 6 hours after the animals had been exposed to isoflurane or halothane. Furthermore, the iNOS inhibitor aminoguanidine eliminated the infarct-sparing effect of anesthetic preconditiononing (Kapinya et al., 2002).

3.2. Remote Cytokine Responses

Cellular responses to focal ischemia are not restricted to the ischemic lesion, but also involve the non-ischemic remote cortex. Microglia transiently up-regulated complement receptor-3 (CR-3), an immunological indicator for their activation, and cortical astrocytes responded by expressing higher levels of GFAP (Schroeter et al., 1995; Schroeter et al., 1999; Yamashita et al., 1996). This glial activation peaked between day 3 and 7. In remote neurons, the inflammatory enzyme cyclooxygenase (COX)-2 was induced (Miettinen et al., 1997). Most of these changes were observed in the ipsilateral but not contralateral hemisphere and could be blocked by the non-competetive N-methyl-D-aspartate (NMDA) receptor antagonist MK-801. Importantly, brain areas with remote cellular responses after cerebral ischemia were devoid of histologically detectable tissue damage, leukocyte recruitment, and apoptotic cell death (Braun et al., 1996; Isenmann et al., 1998).

Discernible glial activation on morphological grounds is preceded by rapid molecular responses. Within hours a rapid increase in IL-1β and TNF-α mRNA levels could be found in the non-ischemic cortex reaching peak levels within the first 24 hrs (Jander et al., 2000). On the protein level, IL-1β was expressed by cortical microglia within 4 hrs and normalized at 16 hrs (Jander et al., 2001). The cellular origin of TNF-α is unclear at present although some evidence suggests that it is produced by neurons. Interestingly, remote IL-1β and TNF-α responses were not paralleled by an increase in iNOS mRNA levels, which is in contrast to the expression pattern found within the ischemic core. Cytokine-mediated exacerbation of excitotoxic neuronal cell death in vitro depends on the expression of iNOS (Hewett et al., 1994). The co-expression of TNF-α, IL-1β and iNOS in ischemic brain areas may therefore mediate secondary expansion of the infarct as shown in iNOS-deficient mice (Iadecola et al., 1997b) (see also section 3.1.4.). Contrastingly in the absence of iNOS activity, both TNF-α and IL-1β may save neurons from hypoxic and excitotoxic damage (Cheng et al., 1994; Strijbos and Rothwell, 1995) and confer neuroprotection. Remote IL-1β induction after focal ischemia, moreover, appears to be involved in postischemic brain plasticity. Schneider et al. (1998) could demonstrate that IL-1β contributes to the maintenance of long-term potentiation (LTP) without affecting its induction. LTP plays an important role in brain plasticity and is facilitated in close vicinity of ischemic brain lesions (Hagemann et al., 1998).

Remote cytokine responses after focal cerebral ischemia could completely be blocked by MK-801 application. This indicates that glutaminergic signalling through NMDA-receptors is involved (Jander et al., 2000). It has been known for several years that focal ischemic brain lesions in rodents trigger periinfarct depolarizations that closely resemble cortical spreading depression (CSD) (Schroeter et al., 1995; Dietrich et al., 1994). CSD is characterized by a transient suppression of all neuronal activity that repetitively extends from sites of increased extracellular potassium concentrations to the entire ipsilateral hemisphere, while the contralateral cortex is spared (Martins Ferreira et al., 2000). CSD can be blocked by MK-801 (Lauritzen and Hansen, 1992). Isolated CSD by focal application of KCl to the brain surface induces a similar cytokine response as observed in remote cortex after focal ischemia (Jander et al., 2001). In the normal brain, CSD mediates neuronal tolerance against a subsequent lethal ischemic challenge (Kobayashi et al., 1995; Yanamoto, et al., 1998) while in the ischemic brain energy consuming CSD may be involved in the expansion of the infarct core into the ischemic penumbra (Hossmann, 1994)

4. Inflammation and Neuroprotection

4.1. Immune Tolerance and Neuroprotection

Cellular infiltration after ischemia has mainly been studied under the hypothesis of a detrimental role in infarct development. Recently a novel concept emerged suggesting that inflammation in the nervous system may also be beneficial and neuroprotection to ischemic damage can be achieved by manipulating the immune system.

Immune tolerance is defined as the specific suppression of cellular and/or humoral immune responses to an antigen by prior administration of the antigen (Weiner, 2001). In a more widespread definition immune tolerance describes any mechanism by which a potentially injurious immune response is prevented, suppressed, or shifted. Mucosal tolerance is a well-established model whereby immunological tolerance is induced to a specific antigen through nasal instillation or feeding (Weiner, 1997; Metzler and Wraith, 1996). Antigen administered nasally or orally encounters the respective mucosa-associated lymphoid tissue, which forms a well developed immune network. On antigen re-stimulation, T cells tolerized with a low-dose regime preferentially secrete IL-10 and IL-4 (Th2-response) or TGF-β (Th3-response) and thereby suppress cell-mediated or TH1 immune responses. Although activation of T cells is specific for the tolerizing antigen, the immunomudulatory cytokines secreted in response to activation have non-specific effects leading to "bystander suppression" (Faria and Weiner, 1999).

Mucosal administration of autoantigens has been primarily shown to suppress inflammation and disease activity in several models of autoimmunity such as diabetes, arthritis, and experimental allergic encephalomyelitis (Faria and Weiner, 1999). However, this approach has also recently been used to treat stroke in experimental animal models. Control of inflammation associated with brain ischemia was achieved by inducing mucosal tolerance to the myelin basic protein (MBP) (Becker et al., 1997; Frenkel et al., 2004). Infarct size at 24, 72 and 96 hrs after MCAO was significantly reduced in tolerized animals. Tolerance to MBP was confirmed in vivo by a decrease in delayed-type hypersensitivity to MBP and immunoreactive TGF-β expression by T cells was found only in the brains of tolerized animals. The neuroprotective effect of MBP tolerization is specifically mediated by CD4+ T cells and IL-10. Adoptive transfer of CD4+ T cells to untreated mice from nasally tolerized animals before MCAO significantly reduced the infarct size, whereas CD4+ T cells from nasally tolerized IL-10-deficient mice had no effect (Frenkel et al., 2004). Taken together, these results emphasize that MBP-specific deviation of the immune response towards TH2 or TH3 lymphocytes has a neuroprotective effect in animal models of ischemic stroke. Takeda et al. (2002) investigated the effect of mucosal tolerance to human E-selectin for stroke prevention in spontaneously hypertensive stroke-prone rats. The rationale of this approach is to target regulatory T cells to vessels that are becoming activated. Since E-selectin is only expressed on activated endothelium it stimulates local production of immunosuppressive cytokines such as TGF-β1, when locally presented to tolerized T cells. TGF-β1 then suppresses the production of proinflammatory cytokines, reduces endothelial thrombogenicity and minimizes vessel damage. In line with this hypothesis, intranasal E-selectin indeed decreased the number and size of ischemic and hemorrhagic strokes in spontaneously hypertensive stroke-prone rats. Furthermore, it suppressed delayed-type hypersensitivity to E-selectin and increased the number of TGF-β1-positive splenocytes. In contrast to the available immunosuppressive agents which have systemic side effects that limit their long-term use in the prevention of stroke, the mucosal administration of proteins offers the potential for long-term antigen-specific therapy that targets regulatory cells to the disease area without systemic immunosuppression.

4.2. Pre-Conditioning, Cytokines and Neuroprotection

When applied below the threshold of injury, virtually any stimulus can activate endogenous protective mechanisms in the brain, which mitigate the damage from consecutive severe stress (Dirnagl et al., 2003). As an example patients with ipsilateral transient ischemic attacks occurring shorty before a manifest cortical infarct developed statistically smaller infarcts (Weih et al., 1999; Moncayo et al., 2000; Castillo et al., 2003). In the experimental setting several molecular pathways of ischemic pre-conditioning have been elucidated. Lipopolysaccharide (LPS) as a bacterial antigen represents the prototypic stimulus for cytokine induction. Administration of LPS effectively protected various organs against subsequent ischemic damage. In the brain, intraperitoneal LPS injection 72 hrs before transient MCAO reduced brain infarct volume by 35 % compared to controls. This effect was associated with an increase of superoxide dismutase and eNOS expression (Bordet et al., 2000; Puisieux et al, 2000). In an excitotoxic brain lesion model in the mouse using kainic acid, LPS pre-conditioning 24 hrs before the "true" lesion afforded neuroprotection to CA3 neurons in the hippocampus (Boche et al., 2003). Further investigations on the underlying mechanisms revealed increased TGF-β1 and IL-1β levels after the administration of LPS.

The proinflammatory cytokines IL-1 and TNF-α, which are robustly up-regulated by LPS, have also been shown to induce tolerance to brain ischemia. IL-1 pre-conditioning in a global ischemia model in gerbils saved CA1 hippocampal neurons from severe ischemia and this effect could be blocked by IL-1ra (Ohtsuki et al., 1996). TNF is regarded as an "alarm hormone" that is ubiquitously produced in response to stress. Intravenous pre-treatment of rats with LPS led to the development of ischemic tolerance, an effect that could be prevented by co-administration of TNF-α-binding protein (Tasaki et al., 1997). In addition, ischemic preconditioning mediated up-regulation of TNF-α and induced the expression of TNF-α convertase (TACE) in vitro and in vivo (Liu et al., 2000; Cardenas et al., 2002; Romera et al., 2004). Intracisternal administration of TNF-α protected animals from ischemic injury after permanent MCAO (Nawashiro et al., 1997) and mice mutants lacking TNF receptors developed larger infarcts after focal cerebral ischemia, which is in further support of a neuroptrotective role of TNF-α (Bruce et al., 1996; Gary et al., 1998). The molecular mechanisms of TNF-α mediated neuroprotection are not yet fully understood, but the induction of Ca2+ scavenger proteins and mangane-superoxide dismutase are probably involved (Mattson, 1997). Ischemic tolerance that developed with a delay of 24-72 hrs was accompanied by TNF-α mediated ceramide expression. Under certain conditions, ceramide serves as a cytoprotectant (Goodman and Mattson, 1996) and the intraventricular application of ceramide reduced neuronal damage after hypoxia-ischemia in new-born rats (Chen et al.,

2001). Therapeutic effects of ceramide were paralleled by an induction of bcl-2 molecules, which act anti-apoptotic. In line with this result, a reduced number of apoptotic cells were found within the lesions. Taken together, present data suggest that TNF-α is harmful in the acute phase of cerebral ischemia (see also section 3.1.2.), but these negative effects are counteracted by an essential role of TNF-α-mediated in neuroprotection, recovery and repair.

Besides the above mentioned proinflammatory cytokines, antiinflammatory molecules are likewise up-regulated after focal cerebral ischemia. Increased levels of IL-10 mRNA have been found six hrs after MCAO in rodents (Zhai et al., 1997). Furthermore, local or systemic administration of IL-10 significantly reduced infarct volumes after transient MCAO (Spera et al., 1998) when treatment was applied within 30 minutes after stroke onset. In line with a neuroprotective role of IL-10, IL-10 knock out mice developed 30 % larger infarcts compared to control animals (Grilli et al., 2000). The beneficial effects of IL-10 in experimental ischemic stroke could either be mediated by the attenuation of the inflammatory cascade and/or the inhibition of neurotoxic signalling. IL-10, when administered exogenously, inhibits the transcription of TNF and NFκB. Moreover, primary neuronal cultures derived from IL-10 null mutants were more susceptible to excitotoxicity and oxygen-glucose deprivation (Grilli et al., 2000) and IL-10 diminished glutamate-induced cerebellar granule cell death in vitro via the blockade of casapse-3-like activity (Bachis et al., 2001). A recent clinical study provides first evidence for a possible role of IL-10 in stroke prevention in humans. In this trial which enrolled 599 subjects $\geq$ 85 years (Van Exel et al., 2002) patients with a history of stroke had significantly lower IL-10 serum levels than subjects without former cerebral ischemia. During the follow-up period of 2.6 years, the relative risk for fatal stroke was 2.94 when subjects with low or intermediate baseline IL-10 production were compared to those with high IL-10 levels. It appeared that a relative IL-10 deficiency bears an increased stroke risk of stroke even in a healthy population. At present it is a matter of debate whether this effect is related to a potentially protective role of IL-10 in atherogenesis rather than affecting the brain parenchyma directly.

Transforming growth factor-β1 (TGF-β1) is another primarily antiinflammatory cytokine with neuroprotective abilities. TGF-β1 is involved in the regulation of numerous cellular processes: It maintains the mitochondrial membrane potential, stabilizes Ca2+ homeostasis and increases the expression of the anti-apoptotic proteins Bcl-2 and Bcl-xl (Prehn et al., 1998). During the first week after focal cerebral ischemia TGF-β1 expression associated with microglia and infiltrating macrophages subsequently increases and parallels the induction of IL-18 (Lehrmann et al., 1998; Stoll et al., 2004). Functionally, TGF-β1 had beneficial effects on glutamate-induced excitotoxic cell death in neuronal cell culture systems suggesting a physiological role as a neuroprotectant in CNS lesions (Prehn et al., 1998; Ruocco et al., 1999). This hypothesis is supported by neutralization experiments. Application of a soluble TGF-β type II receptor fused with the Fc region of human immunoglobulin thereby neutralizing endogenous TGF-β1 in rats subjected to MCAO strongly aggravated ischemic brain damage (Ruocco et al., 1999). In another study in rats, TGF-β1 reduced damage to CA1 hippocampal neurons caused by transient global ischemia (Henrich-Noack et al., 1996). A slightly mitigating effect was present after MCAO in mice that had received TGF-β1 intracisternally (Prehn et al., 1998). In addition, TGF-β1 injection to the lateral ventricle of rats 2 hrs after severe hypoxic-ischemic brain injury reduced the volume of cortical infarction

(McNeill et al., 1994). Taken together, these findings suggest that endogenous TGF-β1 limits the extent of brain injury after stroke and that additionally administered exogenous TGF-β1 is able to support neuroprotection, at least to some degree. In humans, published data on TGF-β in stroke are inconclusive. Kim et al (1996) reported decreased TGF-β serum levels at day 1 and day 3 after cerebral ischemia while others did not find significant differences between serum TGF-β levels from patients and controls at any time point (Slevin et al., 2000).

4.3. Hematopoietic Growth Factors and Neuroprotection

4.3.1. Erythropoietin

Besides cytokines, hematopoietic growth factors have recently been shown to mediate neuroprotection in brain hypoxia and focal cerebral ischemia (Brines and Cerami, 2005). The glycoprotein hormone erythropoietin (EPO) was originally discovered as a kidney-derived stimulator of erythroid progenitor cell proliferation and differentiation (Bauer, 1995). EPO is in clinical use to treat patients with severe anemia. EPO gene expression in most tissues, including brain, is regulated by the transcription factor, hypoxia-inducible factor-1 (HIF-1) that is activated by a variety of stressors, including hypoxia (Jelkmann, 1994; Ebert and Bunn, 1999). Low EPO and EPO receptor (EPOr) levels are expressed in rodent and human brain tissue under non-pathological conditions. Neurons and astrocytes appear to be the main cellular sources (Marti et al., 1996; Juul et al., 1999; Siren et al., 2001a; Bernaudin et al., 1999). In hippocampal neuronal cultures both EPO and EPOr were induced by hypoxia (Lewczuk et al., 2000). In vivo, rats subjected to two hrs of hypoxia likewise displayed increased EPO and EPOr expression in the hippocampus (Siren and Ehrenreich, 2001b). Prass and colleagues (2003) recently demonstrated that hypoxia-induced stroke tolerance is specifically mediated by EPO. In their study hypoxic pre-conditioning for 180 to 300 minutes induced relative tolerance to transient focal cerebral ischemia, as evidenced by a reduction of infarct volumes by 54% to 75% of the control, respectively. Sixty minutes after brain hypoxia a marked activation of HIF-1 DNA-binding activity and a 7-fold induction of EPO transcription was found and the infusion of soluble EPOr significantly reduced the protective effect of hypoxic pre-treatment by 40%. In the acute phase after experimental cerebral ischemia EPO expression was linked to endothelial cells (day 1). Subsequently, its expression shifted to microglia/macrophage-like cells (day 3) and was finally found in reactive astrocytes at later stages of infarct development (day 7) (Sadamoto et al., 1998; Bernaudin et al., 1999). EPOr expression always preceded the induction of EPO for each cell type indicating that there is continuous formation of EPO with its corresponding receptor during the evolution of ischemic stroke. In vitro, exogenously administered EPO protected cultured cortical neurons from oxygen-glucose deprivation and AMPA/NMDA-receptor mediated excitotoxicity (Sinor and Greenberg, 2000; Sakanaka et al, 1998). Using models of experimental cerebral ischemia several studies have demonstrated that EPO is able to reduce infarct size and neurological deficits in vivo (Brines et al., 2000; Siren et al., 2001c; Leist et al., 2004). Functionally, EPO rescues neurons within the penumbra from apoptosis (Siren et al., 2001c), reduces the activation of astrocytes and microglia and decreases the production of pro-inflammatory cytokines, e. g. TNF, IL-6 and MCP-1 (Villa et al., 2003).

Siren et al. (2001a) recently investigated the distribution of EPO immunoreactivity in human brain sections after ischemia and/or hypoxia. Acutely after stroke (< 5 days), EPO was found in vascular tissue and inflammatory cells, while EPOr was located to blood vessels and neuronal as well as astrocytic cell processes within the infarcts and the periinfarct zone. In older ischemic infarctions (< 18 days) EPO and its receptor were strongest in reactive glia. Acute hypoxic brain damage was associated with strong EPO expression in blood vessels while the EPOr was mainly found in neuronal processes. A previously published phase I clinical trial investigated the safety and efficacy of recombinant EPO in patients with ischemic stroke within the middle cerebral artery territory (Ehrenreich et al., 2002). The time window between the onset of symptoms and the administration of the study drug was < 8 hrs and EPO was applied intravenously. Overall, no safety concerns were identified in 13 patients participating in the safety part of the study. EPO treatment in the efficacy part (40 patients) was associated with an improvement in follow-up and neurological outcome scales. However, reduction of infarct size in EPO-treated patients compared to controls was statistically not significant, although a strong trend towards smaller infarcts was observed.

4.3.2. Granulocyte Colony Stimulating Factor

Granulocyte colony stimulating factor (G-CSF) is another member of the glycoprotein growth factor family with neuroprotective properties. G-CSF mainly controls the survival, proliferation and differentiation of hematopoietic progenitor cells, but also activates neutrophils and monocytes (Boneberg and Hartung, 2002). Only recently, the profound anti-inflammatory properties of G-CSF have been disclosed: (i) in vitro, G-CSF down-regulated LPS-stimulated TNF expression in monocytes (Boneberg and Hartung, 2002), and (ii) in vivo, G-CSF reduced TNF expression during experimental autoimmune encephalomyelitis, a model for human multiple sclerosis, and inflammation-associated tissue damage (Zavala et al., 2002). In the normal brain, G-CSF is constitutively expressed by neurons (Kleinschnitz et al., 2004b). Within 4 hrs after focal cerebral ischemia G-CSF gene expression is massively up-regulated. Thus, G-CSF may act as an intrinsic neuroprotectant. Functionally, administration of exogenous G-CSF exerted neuroprotective effects in a cell culture model of glutamate-mediated neurotoxicity and reduced infarct volumes after MCAO in vivo without increasing the number of infiltrating neutrophils (Schäbitz et al., 2003; Six et al., 2003). In a recent study by Shyu and colleagues (2004), rats receiving subcutaneous G-CSF showed less cerebral infarction and improved motor performance compared to sham-treated animals. Furthermore, G-CSF enhanced the availability of circulating hematopoietic stem cells to the brain and their capacity for neurogenesis and angiogenesis in the ischemic region (Schneider et al., 2005). Consequently, G-CSF and other hematopoietic growth factors are recently tested in several clinical trials in stroke and other neurological diseases but available data are too limited yet to draw any firm conclucsions concerning their safety or efficacy (Bath and Sprigg, 2007).

REFERENCES

Alexander M, Forster C, Sugimoto K, Clark HB, Vogel S, Ross ME, Iadecola C (2003). Interferon regulatory factor-1 immunoreactivity in neurons and inflammatory cells following ischemic stroke in rodents and humans. *Acta Neuropathol 105*, 420-424.

Allen SM, Rothwell NJ (2001). Cytokines and acute neurodegeneration. *Nature Reviews Neuroscience 2*, 734-744.

Arai KI, Lee F, Miyajima A, Miyatake S, Arai N, Yokota T (1990). Cytokines: coordinators of immune and inflammatory responses. *Annu Rev Biochem 59*, 783-836.

Arumugam TV, Salter JW, Chidlow JH, Ballantyne CM, Kevil CG, Granger DN (2004) Contributions of LFA-1 and Mac-1 to brain injury and microvascular dysfunction induced by transient middle cerebral artery occlusion. *Am J Physiol Heart Circ Physiol 287*, H2555-2560.

Arvin B, Neville LF, Barone FC, Feuerstein GZ (1996). The role of inflammation and cytokines in brain injury. *Neurosci Biobehav Rev 20*, 445-452.

Bachis A, Colangelo AM, Vicini S, Doe PP, De Bernardi MA, Brooker G, Mocchetti I (2001). Interleukin-10 prevents glutamate-mediated cerebellar granule cell death by blocking caspase-3-like activity. *J Neurosci 21*, 3104-3112.

Barone FC, Arvin B, White RF, Miller A, Webb CL, Willette RN, Lysko PG, Feuerstein GZ (1997). Tumor necrosis factor-alpha. A mediator of focal ischemic brain injury. *Stroke 28*, 1233-1244.

Bath PM, Sprigg N (2007) Colony stimulating factors (including erythropoietin, granulocyte colony stimulating factor and analogues) for stroke. *Cochrane Database Syst Rev 2*, CD005207.

Bauer C (1995). Erythropoietin--from gene structure to therapeutic applications. *J Perinat Med 23*, 77-81.

Becker KJ, McCarron RM, Ruetzler C, Laban O, Sternberg E, Flanders KC, Hallenbeck JM (1997). Immunologic tolerance to myelin basic protein decreases stroke size after transient focal cerebral ischemia. *Proc Natl Acad Sci U S A 94*, 10873-10878.

Bendszus M, Stoll G (2003). Caught in the act: in vivo mapping of macrophage infiltration in nerve injury by magnetic resonance imaging. *J Neurosci 23*, 10892-10896.

Bernaudin M, Marti HH, Roussel S, Divoux D, Nouvelot A, MacKenzie ET, Petit E (1999). A potential role for erythropoietin in focal permanent cerebral ischemia in mice. *J Cereb Blood Flow Metab 19*, 643-651.

Bhat RV, DiRocco R, Marcy VR, Flood DG, Zhu Y, Dobrzanski P, Siman R, Scott R, Contreras PC, Miller M (1996). Increased expression of IL-1beta converting enzyme in hippocampus after ischemia: selective localization in microglia. *J Neurosci 16*, 4146-4154.

Boche D, Cunningham C, Gauldie J, Perry VH (2003). Transforming growth factor-beta 1-mediated neuroprotection against excitotoxic injury in vivo. *J Cereb Blood Flow Metab 23*, 1174-1182.

Boneberg EM, Hartung T (2002). Molecular aspects of anti-inflammatory action of G-CSF. *Inflamm Res 51*, 119-128.

Bordet R, Deplanque D, Maboudou P, Puisieux F, Pu Q, Robin E, Martin A, Bastide M, Leys D, Lhermitte M, Dupuis B (2000). Increase in endogenous brain superoxide dismutase as a potential mechanism of lipopolysaccharide-induced brain ischemic tolerance. *J Cereb Blood Flow Metab 20*, 1190-1196.

Botchkina GI, Meistrell ME 3rd, Botchkina IL, Tracey KJ (1997). Expression of TNF and TNF receptors (p55 and p75) in the rat brain after focal cerebral ischemia. *Mol Med 3*, 765-781.

Boutin H, LeFeuvre RA, Horai R, Asano M, Iwakura Y, Rothwell NJ (2001). Role of IL-1alpha and IL-1beta in ischemic brain damage. *J Neurosci 21*, 5528-5534.

Braun JS, Jander S, Schroeter M, Witte OW, Stoll G (1996). Spatiotemporal relationship of apoptotic cell death to lymphomonocytic infiltration in photochemically induced focal ischemia of the rat cerebral cortex. *Acta Neuropathol 92*, 255-263.

Brines ML, Ghezzi P, Keenan S, Agnello D, de Lanerolle NC, Cerami C, Itri LM, Cerami A (2000). Erythropoietin crosses the blood-brain barrier to protect against experimental brain injury. *Proc Natl Acad Sci U S A 97*, 10526-10531.

Brines M, Cerami A (2005) Emerging biological roles for erythropoietin in the nervous system. Nat Rev Neurosci. 2005 Jun;6(6):484-94.

Bruce AJ, Boling W, Kindy MS, Peschon J, Kraemer PJ, Carpenter MK, Holtsberg FW, Mattson MP (1996). Altered neuronal and microglial responses to excitotoxic and ischemic brain injury in mice lacking TNF receptors. *Nat Med 2*, 788-794.

Buttini M, Sauter A, Boddeke HW (1994). Induction of interleukin-1 beta mRNA after focal cerebral ischaemia in the rat. *Brain Res Mol Brain Res 23*, 126-134.

Cardenas A, De Alba J, Moro MA, Leza JC, Lorenzo P, Lizasoain I (1998). Protective effect of N-(3-(aminomethyl)benzyl) acetamidine, an inducible nitric oxide synthase inhibitor, in brain slices exposed to oxygen-glucose deprivation. *Eur J Pharmacol 354*, 161-165.

Cardenas A, Moro MA, Leza JC, O'Shea E, Davalos A, Castillo J, Lorenzo P, Lizasoain I (2002). Upregulation of TACE/ADAM17 after ischemic preconditioning is involved in brain tolerance. *J Cereb Blood Flow Metab 22*, 1297-1302.

Castillo J, Moro MA, Blanco M, Leira R, Serena J, Lizasoain I, Davalos A (2003). The release of tumor necrosis factor-alpha is associated with ischemic tolerance in human stroke. *Ann Neurol 54*, 811-819.

Chen F, Ward J, Robinson PJ (1999). MR imaging of the liver and spleen: a comparison of the effects on signal intensity of two superparamagnetic iron oxide agents. *Magn Reson Imaging 17*, 549-556.

Chen Y, Ginis I, Hallenbeck JM (2001). The protective effect of ceramide in immature rat brain hypoxia-ischemia involves up-regulation of bcl-2 and reduction of TUNEL-positive cells. *J Cereb Blood Flow Metab 21*, 34-40.

Cheng B, Christakos S, Mattson MP (1994). Tumor necrosis factors protect neurons against metabolic-excitotoxic insults and promote maintenance of calcium homeostasis. *Neuron 12*, 139-153.

Chopp M, Li Y, Jiang N, Zhang RL, Prostak J (1996). Antibodies against adhesion molecules reduce apoptosis after middle cerebral artery occlusion in rats. *J Cereb Blood Flow Metabol 16*, 578-584.

Connolly ES, Winfree CJ, Springer TA, Naka Y, Yan SD, Stern DM, Solomon RA, Gutlererez-Ramos JC, Pinski DJ (1996). Cerebral protection in homozygous null ICAM-1 mice after middle cerebral artery occlusion: role of neutrophil adhesion in the pathogenesis of stroke. *J Clin Invest 97*, 209-216.

Dalkara T, Yoshida T, Irikura K, Moskowitz MA (1994). Dual role of nitric oxide in focal cerebral ischemia. *Neuropharmacology 33*, 1447-1452.

De Alba J, Cardenas A, Moro MA, Leza JC, Lorenzo P, Bosca L, Lizasoain I (1999). Down-regulation of neuronal nitric oxide synthase by nitric oxide after oxygen-glucose deprivation in rat forebrain slices. *J Neurochem 72*, 248-254.

Del Zoppo G, Ginis I, Hallenbeck JM, Iadecola C, Wang X, Feuerstein GZ (2000). Inflammation and stroke: putative role for cytokines, adhesion molecules and iNOS in brain response to ischemia. *Brain Pathol 10*, 95-112.

Dietrich D, Feng ZC, Leistra H, Watson BD, Rosenthal M (1994). Photothrombotic infarction triggers multiple episodes of cortical spreading depression in distant brain regions. *J Cereb Blood Flow Metab 14*, 20-28.

Dirnagl U, Iadecola C, Moskowitz MA (1999). Pathobiology of ischaemic stroke: an integrated view. *Trends Neurosci. 22*, 391-397.

Dirnagl U, Simon RP, Hallenbeck JM (2003). Ischemic tolerance and endogenous neuroprotection. *Trends Neurosci 26*, 248-254.

Ebert BL, Bunn HF (1999). Regulation of the erythropoietin gene. *Blood 94*, 1864-1877.

Ehrenreich H, Hasselblatt M, Dembowski C, Cepek L, Lewczuk P, Stiefel M, Rustenbeck HH, Breiter N, Jacob S, Knerlich F, Bohn M, Poser W, Ruther E, Kochen M, Gefeller O, Gleiter C, Wessel TC, De Ryck M, Itri L, Prange H, Cerami A, Brines M, Siren AL (2002). Erythropoietin therapy for acute stroke is both safe and beneficial. *Mol Med 8*, 495-505.

Endoh M, Maiese K, Wagner J (1994). Expression of the inducible form of nitric oxide synthase by reactive astrocytes after transient global ischemia. *Brain Res 651*, 92-100.

Enlimomab Acute Stroke Trial Investigators (2001). Use of anti-ICAM-1 therapy in ischemic stroke. *Neurology 57*, 1428-1434.

Faria AM, Weiner HL (1999). Oral tolerance: mechanisms and therapeutic applications. *Adv Immunol 73*, 153-264.

Ferriero DM, Holtzman DM, Black SM, Sheldon RA (1996). Neonatal mice lacking neuronal nitric oxide synthase are less vulnerable to hypoxic-ischemic injury. *Neurobiol Dis 3*, 64-71.

Feuerstein GZ, Liu T, Barone FC (1994). Cytokines, inflammation, and brain injury: role of tumor necrosis factor-alpha. *Cerebrovasc Brain Metab Rev 6*, 341-360.

Flaris NA, Densmore TL, Molleston MC, Hickey WF (1993). Characterization of microglia and macrophages in the central nervous system of rats: definition of the differential expression of molecules using standard and novel monoclonal antibodies in normal CNS and in four models of parenchymal reaction. *Glia 7*, 34-40.

Frederix K, Chauhan AK, Kisucka J, Zhao BQ, Hoff EI, Spronk HM, Ten Cate H, Wagner DD (2007) Platelet adhesion receptors do not modulate infarct volume after a photochemically induced stroke in mice. *Brain Res*, doi:10.1016/j.brainres.2007.07.103.

Frenkel D, Huang Z, Maron R, Koldzic DN, Hancock WW, Moskowitz MA, Weiner HL (2004). Nasal vaccination with myelin oligodendrocyte glycoprotein reduces stroke size by inducing IL-10-producing CD4+ T cells. *J Immunol 171*, 6549-6555.

Furlan M, Marchal G, Viader F, Deerlon JM, Baron JC (1996). Spontaneous neurological recovery after stroke and the fate of the ischemic penumbra. *Ann Neurol 40*, 216-226.

Garcia JH, Yoshida Y, Chen H, Li Y, Zhang ZG, Lian J, Chen S, Chopp M (1993). Progression from ischemic injury to infarct following middle cerebral artery occlusion in the rat. *Am J Pathol 142*, 623-635.

Garcia JH, Liu KF, Yoshida Y, Lian J, Chen S, del Zoppo G (1994). Influx of leukocytes and platelets in an evolving brain infarct (Wistar rat). *Am J Pathol 144*, 188-199.

Garcia JH, Liu KF, Relton JK (1995). Interleukin-1 receptor antagonist decreases the number of necrotic neurons in rats with middle cerebral artery occlusion. *Am J Pathol 147*, 1477-1486.

Gary DS, Bruce-Keller AJ, Kindy MS, Mattson MP (1998). Ischemic and excitotoxic brain injury is enhanced in mice lacking the p55 tumor necrosis factor receptor. *J Cereb Blood Flow Metab 18*, 1283-1287.

Gerriets T, Stolz E, Walberer M, Müller C, Rottger C, Kluge A, Kaps M, Fisher M, Bachmann G (2004). Complications and pitfalls in rat stroke models for middle cerebral artery occlusion. *Stroke 35*, 2372-2377.

Gibson CL, Coughlan TC, Murphy SP (2005) Glial nitric oxide and ischemia. *Glia 50*, 417-426.

Gillen C, Jander S, Stoll G (1998). Sequential expression of mRNA for proinflammatory cytokines and interleukin-10 in the rat peripheral nervous system: comparison between immune-mediated demyelination and Wallerian degeneration. *J Neurosci Res 51*, 489-496.

Ginsberg MD and Busto R (1989). Rodent models of cerebral ischemia. *Stroke 20*, 1627-1642.

Goodman Y, Mattson MP (1996). Ceramide protects hippocampal neurons against excitotoxic and oxidative insults, and amyloid beta-peptide toxicity. *J Neurochem 66*, 869-872.

Gourmala NG, Buttini M, Limonta S, Sauter A, Boddeke HW (1997). Differential and time-dependent expression of monocyte chemoattractant protein-1 mRNA by astrocytes and macrophages in rat brain: effects of ischemia and peripheral lipopolysaccharide administration. *J Neuroimmunol 74*, 35-44.

Goyagi T, Goto S, Bhardwaj A, Dawson VL, Hurn PD, Kirsch JR (2001). Neuroprotective effect of sigma(1)-receptor ligand 4-phenyl-1-(4-phenylbutyl) piperidine (PPBP) is linked to reduced neuronal nitric oxide production. *Stroke 32*, 1613-1620.

Grandati M, Verrecchia C, Revaud ML, Allix M, Boulu RG, Plotkine M (1997). Calcium-independent NO-synthase activity and nitrites/nitrates production in transient focal cerebral ischaemia in mice. *Br J Pharmacol 122*, 625-630.

Gregersen R, Lambertsen K, Finsen B (2000). Microglia and macrophages are the major source of tumor necrosis factor in permanent middle cerebral artery occlusion in mice. *J Cereb Blood Flow Metab 20*, 53-65.

Grilli M, Barbieri I, Basudev H, Brusa R, Casati C, Lozza G, Ongini E (2000). Interleukin-10 modulates neuronal threshold of vulnerability to ischaemic damage. *Eur J Neurosci 12*, 2265-2272.

Hagemann G, Redecker C, Neumann-Haefelin T, Freund HJ, Witte OW (1998). Increased long-term potentiation in the surround of experimentally induced focal cortical infarction. *Ann Neurol 44*, 255-25s8.

Hara H, Friedlander RM, Gagliardini V, Ayata C, Fink K, Huang Z, Shimizu-Sasamata M, Yuan J, Moskowitz MA (1997). Inhibition of interleukin 1beta converting enzyme family proteases reduces ischemic and excitotoxic neuronal damage. *Proc Natl Acad Sci U S A 94*, 2007-2012.

Hedtjarn M, Leverin AL, Eriksson K, Blomgren K, Mallard C, Hagberg H (2002). Interleukin-18 involvement in hypoxic-ischemic brain injury. *J Neurosci 22*, 5910-59.

Henrich-Noack P, Prehn JH, Krieglstein J (1996). TGF-beta 1 protects hippocampal neurons against degeneration caused by transient global ischemia. Dose-response relationship and potential neuroprotective mechanisms. *Stroke 27*, 1609-1614.

Hewett SJ, Csernansky CA, Choi DW (1994). Selective potentiation of NMDA-induced neuronal injury following induction of astrocytic iNOS. *Neuron 13*, 487-494.

Hirji N, Lin TJ, Bissonnette E, Belosevic M, Befus AD (1998). Mechanisms of macrophage stimulation through CD8: macrophage CD8alpha and CD8beta induce nitric oxide production and associated killing of the parasite Leishmania major. *J Immunol 160*, 6004-6011.

Hossmann KA (1994). Viability thresholds and the penumbra of focal ischemia. *Ann Neurol 36*, 557-565.

Huang Z, Huang PL, Panahian N, Dalkara T, Fishman MC, Moskowitz MA (1994). Effects of cerebral ischemia in mice deficient in neuronal nitric oxide synthase. *Science 265*, 1883-1885.

Huang Z, Huang PL, Ma J, Meng W, Ayata C, Fishman MC, Moskowitz MA (1996). Enlarged infarcts in endothelial nitric oxide synthase knockout mice are attenuated by nitro-L-arginine. *J Cereb Blood Flow Metab 16*, 981-987.

Hurn PD, Subramanian S, Parker SM, Afentoulis ME, Kaler LJ, Vandenbark AA, Offner H (2007) T- and B-cell-deficient mice with experimental stroke have reduced lesion size and inflammation. *J Cereb Blood Flow Metab 27*, 1798-1805.

Iadecola C, Zhang F, Xu S, Casey R, Ross ME (1995a). Inducible nitric oxide synthase gene expression in brain following cerebral ischemia. *J Cereb Blood Flow Metab 15*, 378-384.

Iadecola C, Li J, Ebner TJ, Xu X (1995b). Nitric oxide contributes to functional hyperemia in cerebellar cortex. *Am J Physiol 268*, 1153-1162.

Iadecola C, Zhang F, Casey R, Clark HB, Ross ME (1996). Inducible nitric oxide synthase gene expression in vascular cells after transient focal cerebral ischemia. *Stroke 27*, 1373-1380.

Iadecola C (1997a). Bright and dark sides of nitric oxide in ischemic brain injury. *Trends Neurosci 20*, 132-139.

Iadecola C, Zhang F, Casey R, Nagayama M, Ross ME (1997b). Delayed reduction of ischemic brain injury and neurological deficits in mice lacking the inducible nitric oxide synthase gene. *J Neurosci 17*, 9157-9164.

Iadecola C, Salkowski CA, Zhang F, Aber T, Nagayama M, Vogel SN, Ross ME (1999). The transcription factor interferon regulatory factor 1 is expressed after cerebral ischemia and contributes to ischemic brain injury. *J Exp Med 189*, 719-727.

Imai F, Suzuki H, Oda J, Ninomiya T, Ono K, Sano H, Sawada M (2007) Neuroprotective effect of exogenous microglia in global brain ischemia. *J Cereb Blood Flow Metab 27*, 488-500.

Isenmann S, Stoll G, Schroeter M, Krajewski S, Reed JC, Bahr M (1998). Differential regulation of Bax, Bcl-2, and Bcl-X proteins in focal cortical ischemia in the rat. *Brain Pathol 8*, 49-62.

Ishikawa M, Vowinkel T, Stokes KY, Arumugam TV, Yilmaz G, Nanda A, Granger DN (2005) CD40/CD40 ligand signaling in mouse cerebral microvasculature after focal ischemia/reperfusion. *Circulation 111*, 1690-1696.

Jander S, Kraemer M, Schroeter M, Witte OW, Stoll G (1995). Lymphocytic infiltration and expression of intercellular adhesion molecule-1 in photochemically induced ischemia of the rat cortex. *J Cereb Blood Flow Metabol 15*, 42-51.

Jander S, Pohl J, Gillen C, Schroeter M, Stoll G (1996). Vascular cell adhesion moelcule-1 mRNA is expressed in immune-mediated and ischemic injury of the rat nervous system. *J Neuroimmunol 70*, 75-80.

Jander S, Schroeter M, D'Urso D, Gillen C, Witte OW, Stoll G (1998a). Focal ischaemia of the rat brain elicits an unusual inflammatory response: early appearance of CD8+ macrophages/microglia. *Eur J Neurosci 10*, 680-688.

Jander S, Pohl J, D'Urso D, Gillen C, Stoll G (1998b). Time course and cellular localization of interleukin-10 mRNA and protein expression in autoimmune inflammation of the rat central nervous system. *Am J Pathol 152*, 975-982.

Jander S, Schroeter M, Stoll G (2000). Role of NMDA receptor signaling in the regulation of inflammatory gene expression after focal brain ischemia. *J Neuroimmunol 109*, 181-187.

Jander S, Schroeter M, Peters O, Witte OW, Stoll G (2001). Cortical spreading depression induces proinflammatory cytokine gene expression in the rat brain. *J Cereb Blood Flow Metab 21*, 218-225.

Jander S, Schroeter M, Stoll G (2002). Interleukin-18 expression after focal ischemia of the rat brain: association with the late-stage inflammatory response. *J Cereb Blood Flow Metab 22*, 62-70.

Jelkmann W (1994). Biology of erythropoietin. *Clin Investig 72*, 3-10.

Juul SE, Yachnis AT, Rojiani AM, Christensen RD (1999). Immunohistochemical localization of erythropoietin and its receptor in the developing human brain. *Pediatr Dev Pathol 2*, 148-158.

Kader A, Frazzini VI, Solomon RA, Trifiletti RR (1993). Nitric oxide production during focal cerebral ischemia in rats. *Stroke 24*, 1709-1716.

Kapinya KJ, Lowl D, Futterer C, Maurer M, Waschke KF, Isaev NK, Dirnagl U (2002). Tolerance against ischemic neuronal injury can be induced by volatile anesthetics and is inducible NO synthase dependent. *Stroke 33*, 1889-1898.

Kennedy MK, Torrance DS, Picha KS, Mohler KM (1992). Analysis of cytokine mRNA expression in the central nervous system of mice with experimental autoimmune encephalomyelitis reveals that IL-10 mRNA expression correlates with recovery. *J Immunol 149*, 2496-2505.

Kim JS, Gautam SC, Chopp M, Zaloga C, Jones ML, Ward PA, Welch KM (1995). Expression of monocyte chemoattractant protein-1 and macrophage inflammatory protein-1 after focal cerebral ischemia in the rat. *J Neuroimmunol 56*, 127-134.

Kim JS, Yoon SS, Kim YH, Ryu JS (1996). Serial measurement of interleukin-6, transforming growth factor-beta, and S-100 protein in patients with acute stroke. *Stroke 27*, 1553-1557.

Kleinschnitz C, Bendszus M, Frank M, Solymosi L, Toyka KV, Stoll G (2003). In vivo monitoring of macrophage infiltration in experimental ischemic brain lesions by magnetic resonance imaging. *J Cereb Blood Flow Metab 23*, 1356-1361.

Kleinschnitz C, Brinkhoff J, Zelenka M, Sommer C, Stoll G (2004a). The extent of cytokine induction in peripheral nerve lesions depends on the mode of injury and NMDA receptor signaling. *J Neuroimmunol 149*, 77-83.

Kleinschnitz C, Schroeter M, Jander S, Stoll G (2004b). Induction of granulocyte colony-stimulating factor mRNA by focal cerebral ischemia and cortical spreading depression. *Brain Res Mol Brain Res 131*, 73-78.

Kleinschnitz C, Stoll G, Bendszus M, Schuh K, Pauer HU, Burfeind P, Renné C, Gailani D, Nieswandt B, Renné T (2006) Targeting coagulation factor XII provides protection from pathological thrombosis in cerebral ischemia without interfering with hemostasis. *J Exp Med* 203, 513-8.

Kleinschnitz C, Pozgajova M, Pham M, Bendszus M, Nieswandt B, Stoll G (2007) Targeting platelets in acute experimental stroke: impact of glycoprotein Ib, VI, and IIb/IIIa blockade on infarct size, functional outcome, and intracranial bleeding. *Circulation 115*, 2323-30.

Kleinschnitz C, Braeuninger S, Pham M, Austinat M, Nölte I, Renné T, Nieswandt B, Bendszus M, Stoll G Blocking of Platelets or Intrinsic Coagulation Pathway Driven Thrombosis Does Not Prevent Cerebral Infarctions Induced by Photothrombosis. *Stroke*, in press.

Knowles RG, Moncada S (1994). Nitric oxide synthases in mammals. *Biochem J 298*, 249-258.

Kobayashi S, Harris VA, Welsh FA (1995). Spreading depression induces tolerance of cortical neurons to ischemia in rat brain. *J Cereb Blood Flow Metab 15*, 721-727.

Kochanek PM, Hallenbeck JM (1992). Polymorphonuclear leukocytes and monocytes/macrophages in the pathogenesis of cerebral ischemia and stroke. *Stroke 23*, 1367-1379.

Kriz J, Nguyen MD, Julien JP (2002) Minocycline slows disease progression in a mouse model of amyotrophic lateral sclerosis. *Neurobiol Dis 10*, 268-278.

Kriz J, Gowing G, Julien JP (2003) Efficient three-drug cocktail for disease induced by mutant superoxide dismutase. *Ann Neurol 53*, 429-436

Lalancette-Hébert M, Gowing G, Simard A, Weng YC, Kriz J (2007) Selective ablation of proliferating microglial cells exacerbates ischemic injury in the brain. *J Neurosci 27*, 2596-2605.

Lauritzen M, Hansen AJ (1992). The effect of glutamate receptor blockade on anoxic depolarization and cortical spreading depression. *J Cereb Blood Flow Metab 12*, 223-229.

Lawetzky A, Tiefenthaler G, Kubo R, Hunig T (1990). Identification and characterization of rat T cell subpopulations expressing T cell receptors alpha/beta and gamma/delta. *Eur J Immunol 20*, 343-349.

Lecker R, Shohami E, Abramsky O (1999). Daxanabiolol, a novel neuroprotectice drug in experimental focali schemi. *J Neurol Sci 162*, 114-119.

Lehrmann E, Kiefer R, Christensen T, Toyka KV, Zimmer J, Diemer NH, Hartung HP, Finsen B (1998). Microglia and macrophages are major sources of locally produced transforming growth factor-beta1 after transient middle cerebral artery occlusion in rats. *Glia 24*, 437-448.

Leist M, Ghezzi P, Grasso G, Bianchi R, Villa P, Fratelli M, Savino C, Bianchi M, Nielsen J, Gerwien J, Kallunki P, Larsen AK, Helboe L, Christensen S, Pedersen LO, Nielsen M, Torup L, Sager T, Sfacteria A, Erbayraktar S, Erbayraktar Z, Gokmen N, Yilmaz O, Cerami-Hand C, Xie QW, Coleman T, Cerami A, Brines M (2004). Derivatives of erythropoietin that are tissue protective but not erythropoietic. *Science 305*, 239-242.

Lewczuk P, Hasselblatt M, Kamrowski-Kruck H, Heyer A, Unzicker C, Siren AL, Ehrenreich H (2000). Survival of hippocampal neurons in culture upon hypoxia: effect of erythropoietin. *Neuroreport 11*, 3485-3488.

Liu J, Ginis I, Spatz M, Hallenbeck JM (2000). Hypoxic preconditioning protects cultured neurons against hypoxic stress via TNF-alpha and ceramide. *Am J Physiol Cell Physiol 278*, 144-153.

Liu T, McDonnell PC, Young PR, White RF, Siren AL, Hallenbeck JM, Barone FC, Feurestein GZ (1993). Interleukin-1 beta mRNA expression in ischemic rat cortex. *Stroke 24*, 1746-1750.

Liu T, Clark RK, McDonnell PC, Young PR, White RF, Barone FC, Feuerstein GZ (1994). Tumor necrosis factor-alpha expression in ischemic neurons. *Stroke 25*, 1481-1488.

Loddick SA, MacKenzie A, Rothwell NJ (1996). An ICE inhibitor, z-VAD-DCB attenuates ischaemic brain damage in the rat. *Neuroreport 7*, 1465-1468.

Maeda K, Hata R, Hossmann KA (1998) Differences in the cerebrovascular anatomy of C57Black/6 and SV129 mice. *NeuroReport 9*, 1261-1265.

Marchal G, Beaudouin V, Rioux P, de la Sayette V, Le Doze F, Viader F, Derlon JM, Baron JC (1996). Prolonged persistance of substantial volumes of potentially viable brain tissue after stroke: a correlative PET-CT study with voxel-based data analysis. *Stroke 27*, 599-606.

Marti HH, Wenger RH, Rivas LA, Straumann U, Digicaylioglu M, Henn V, Yonekawa Y, Bauer C, Gassmann M (1996). Erythropoietin gene expression in human, monkey and murine brain. *Eur J Neurosci 8*, 666-676.

Martins-Ferreira H, Nedergaard M, Nicholson C (2000). Perspectives on spreading depression. *Brain Res Brain Res Rev 32*, 215-234.

Mattson MP (1997). Neuroprotective signal transduction: relevance to stroke. *Neurosci Biobehav Rev 21*, 193-206.

Matsuoka Y, Kitamura Y, Tooyama I, Kimura H, Taniguchi T (1997). In vivo hypoxia-induced neuronal damage with an enhancement of neuronal nitric oxide synthase immunoreactivity in hippocampus. *Exp Neurol 146*, 57-66.

McNeill H, Williams C, Guan J, Dragunow M, Lawlor P, Sirimanne E, Nikolics K, Gluckman P (1994). Neuronal rescue with transforming growth factor-beta 1 after hypoxic-ischaemic brain injury. *Neuroreport 14*, 901-904.

Mehler MF, Kessler JA (1997). Hematolymphopoietic and inflammatory cytokines in neural development. *Trends Neurosci 20*, 357-365.

Memezawa H, Smith ML, Siesjö BK (1992). Penumbral tissues salvaged by reperfusion following middle cerebral artery occlusion in rats. *Stroke 23*, 552-559.

Merrill JE, Jonakait GM (1995). Interactions of the nervous and immune systems in development, normal brain homeostasis, and disease. *FASEB J 9*, 611-618.

Metzler B, Wraith DC (1996). *Ann N Y Acad Sci 778*, 228-242.

Miettinen S, Fusco FR, Yrjanheikki J, Keinanen R, Hirvonen T, Roivainen R, Narhi M, Hokfelt T, Koistinaho J (1997). Spreading depression and focal brain ischemia induce cyclooxygenase-2 in cortical neurons through N-methyl-D-aspartic acid-receptors and phospholipase A2. *Proc Natl Acad Sci U S A 94*, 6500-6505.

Moncayo J, de Freitas GR, Bogousslavsky J, Altieri M, van Melle G (2000). Do transient ischemic attacks have a neuroprotective effect? *Neurology 54*, 2089-2094.

Morikawa E, Moskowitz MA, Huang Z, Yoshida T, Irikura K, Dalkara T (1994). L-arginine infusion promotes nitric oxide-dependent vasodilation, increases regional cerebral blood flow, and reduces infarction volume in the rat. *Stroke 25*, 429-435.

Moro MA, De Alba J, Leza JC, Lorenzo P, Fernandez AP, Bentura ML, Bosca L, Rodrigo J, Lizasoain I (1998). Neuronal expression of inducible nitric oxide synthase after oxygen and glucose deprivation in rat forebrain slices. *Eur J Neurosci 10*, 445-456.

Nawashiro H, Tasaki K, Ruetzler CA, Hallenbeck JM (1997). TNF-alpha pretreatment induces protective effects against focal cerebral ischemia in mice. *J Cereb Blood Flow Metab 17*, 483-490.

Nedergaard M, Dirnagl U (2005) Role of glial cells in cerebral ischemia. *Glia 50*, 281-286.

Neumann J, Gunzer M, Gutzeit HO, Ullrich O, Reymann KG, Dinkel K (2006) Microglia provide neuroprotection after ischemia. *FASEB J 20*, 714-716.

Nguyen MD, Julien JP, Rivest S (2002) Innate immunity: the missing link in neuroprotection and neurodegeneration? *Nat Rev Neurosci 3*, 216-227.

Offner H, Subramanian S, Parker SM, Wang C, Afentoulis ME, Lewis A, Vandenbark AA, Hurn PD (2006) Splenic atrophy in experimental stroke is accompanied by increased regulatory T cells and circulating macrophages. *J Immunol 176*, 6523-6531.

Ohtsuki T, Ruetzler CA, Tasaki K, Hallenbeck JM (1996). Interleukin-1 mediates induction of tolerance to global ischemia in gerbil hippocampal CA1 neurons. *J Cereb Blood Flow Metab 16*, 1137-1142.

Oprica M, Van Dam AM, Lundkvist J, Iverfeldt K, Winblad B, Bartfai T, Schultzberg M (2004). Effects of chronic overexpression of interleukin-1 receptor antagonist in a model of permanent focal cerebral ischemia in mouse. *Acta Neuropathol 108*, 69-80.

Parmentier S, Bohme GA, Lerouet D, Damour D, Stutzmann JM, Margaill I, Plotkine M (1999). Selective inhibition of inducible nitric oxide synthase prevents ischaemic brain injury. *Br J Pharmacol 127*, 546-552.

Prass K, Scharff A, Ruscher K, Lowl D, Muselmann C, Victorov I, Kapinya K, Dirnagl U, Meisel A (2003). Hypoxia-induced stroke tolerance in the mouse is mediated by erythropoietin. *Stroke 34*, 1981-1986.

Prehn JH, Backhauss C, Krieglstein J (1998). Transforming growth factor-beta 1 prevents glutamate neurotoxicity in rat neocortical cultures and protects mouse neocortex from ischemic injury in vivo. *J Cereb Blood Flow Metab 13*, 521-525.

Prüss H, Prass K, Ghaeni L, Milosevic M, Muselmann C, Freyer D, Royl G, Reuter U, Baeva N, Dirnagl U, Meisel A, Priller J (2007) Inducible nitric oxide synthase does not mediate brain damage after transient focal cerebral ischemia in mice. *J Cereb Blood Flow Metab* doi: 10.1038/sj.jcbfm.9600550

Puisieux F, Deplanque D, Pu Q, Souil E, Bastide M, Bordet R (2000). Differential role of nitric oxide pathway and heat shock protein in preconditioning and lipopolysaccharide-induced brain ischemic tolerance. *Eur J Pharmacol 389*, 71-78.

Rabuffetti M, Sciorati C, Tarozzo G, Clementi E, Manfredi AA, Beltramo M (2000). Inhibition of caspase-1-like activity by Ac-Tyr-Val-Ala-Asp-chloromethyl ketone induces long-lasting neuroprotection in cerebral ischemia through apoptosis reduction and decrease of proinflammatory cytokines. *J Neurosci 20*, 4398-4404.

Relton JK, Rothwell NJ (1992). Interleukin-1 receptor antagonist inhibits ischaemic and excitotoxic neuronal damage in the rat. *Brain Res Bull 29*, 243-246.

Romera C, Hurtado O, Botella SH, Lizasoain I, Cardenas A, Fernandez-Tome P, Leza JC, Lorenzo P, Moro MA (2004). In vitro ischemic tolerance involves upregulation of glutamate transport partly mediated by the TACE/ADAM17-tumor necrosis factor-alpha pathway. *J Neurosci 24*, 1350-1357.

Rothwell NJ, Luheshi GN (2000). Interleukin 1 in the brain: biology, pathology and therapeutic target. *Trends Neurosci 23*, 618-625.

Ruocco A, Nicole O, Docagne F, Ali C, Chazalviel L, Komesli S, Yablonsky F, Roussel S, MacKenzie ET, Vivien D, Buisson A (1999). A transforming growth factor-beta antagonist unmasks the neuroprotective role of this endogenous cytokine in excitotoxic and ischemic brain injury. *J Cereb Blood Flow Metab 19*, 1345-1353.

Rupalla K, Allegrini PR, Sauer D, Wiessner C (1998). Time course of microglia activation and apoptosis in various brain regions after permanent focal cerebral ischemia in mice. *Acta Neuropathol 96*, 172-178.

Sadamoto Y, Igase K, Sakanaka M, Sato K, Otsuka H, Sakaki S, Masuda S, Sasaki R (1998). Erythropoietin prevents place navigation disability and cortical infarction in rats with permanent occlusion of the middle cerebral artery. *Biochem Biophys Res Commun 253*, 26-32.

Sakanaka M, Wen TC, Matsuda S, Masuda S, Morishita E, Nagao M, Sasaki R (1998). In vivo evidence that erythropoietin protects neurons from ischemic damage. *Proc Natl Acad Sci U S A 95*, 4635-4640.

Saleh A, Schroeter M, Jonkmanns C, Hartung HP, Modder U, Jander S (2004). In vivo MRI of brain inflammation in human ischaemic stroke. *Brain 127*, 1670-1677.

Schäbitz WR, Kollmar R, Schwaninger M, Juettler E, Bardutzky J, Scholzke MN, Sommer C, Schwab S (2003). Neuroprotective effect of granulocyte colony-stimulating factor after focal cerebral ischemia. *Stroke 34*, 745-751.

Schneider A, Krüger C, Steigleder T, Weber D, Pitzer C, Laage R, Aronowski J, Maurer MH, Gassler N, Mier W, Hasselblatt M, Kollmar R, Schwab S, Sommer C, Bach A, Kuhn HG, Schäbitz WR (2005) The hematopoietic factor G-CSF is a neuronal ligand that counteracts programmed cell death and drives neurogenesis. *J Clin Invest 115*, 2083-98.

Schneider H, Pitossi F, Balschun D, Wagner A, del Rey A, Besedovsky HO (1998). A neuromodulatory role of interleukin-1beta in the hippocampus. *Proc Natl Acad Sci U S A 95*, 7778-7783.

Schroeter M, Jander S, Witte OW, Stoll G (1994). Local immune responses in the rat cerebral cortex after middle cerebral artery occlusion. *J Neuroimmunol 55*, 195-203.

Schroeter M, Schiene K, Kraemer M, Hagemann G, Weigel H, Eysel UT, Witte OW, Stoll G (1995). Astroglial responses in photochemically induced focal ischemia of the rat cortex. *Exp Brain Res 106*, 1-6.

Schroeter M, Jander S, Witte OW, Stoll G (1999). Heterogeneity of the microglial response in photochemically induced focal ischemia of the rat cerebral cortex. *Neuroscience 89*, 1367-1377.

Schroeter M, Franke C, Stoll G, Hoehn M (2001a). Dynamic changes of MRI abnormalities in relation to inflammation and glial responses after photothrombotic cerebral infarction in the rat brain. *Acta Neuropathol 101*, 114-122.

Schroeter M, Jander S, Huitinga I, Stoll G (2001b). CD8+ phagocytes in focal ischemia of the rat brain: predominant origin from hematogenous macrophages and targeting to areas of pannecrosis. *Acta Neuropathol 101*, 440-448.

Shohami E, Ginis I, Hallenbeck JM (1999). Dual role of tumor necrosis factor alpha in brain injury. *Cytokine Growth Factor Rev 10*, 119-130.

Shyu WC, Lin SZ, Yang HI, Tzeng YS, Pang CY, Yen PS, Li H (2004). Functional recovery of stroke rats induced by granulocyte colony-stimulating factor-stimulated stem cells. *Circulation 110*, 1847-1854.

Sinor AD, Greenberg DA (2000). Erythropoietin protects cultured cortical neurons, but not astroglia, from hypoxia and AMPA toxicity. *Neurosci Lett 290*, 213-215.

Siren AL, Knerlich F, Poser W, Gleiter CH, Bruck W, Ehrenreich H (2001a). Erythropoietin and erythropoietin receptor in human ischemic/hypoxic brain. *Acta Neuropathol 101*, 271-276.

Siren AL, Ehrenreich H (2001b). Erythropoietin--a novel concept for neuroprotection. *Eur Arch Psychiatry Clin Neurosci 251*, 179-184

Siren AL, Fratelli M, Brines M, Goemans C, Casagrande S, Lewczuk P, Keenan S, Gleiter C, Pasquali C, Capobianco A, Mennini T, Heumann R, Cerami A, Ehrenreich H, Ghezzi P (2001c). Erythropoietin prevents neuronal apoptosis after cerebral ischemia and metabolic stress. *Proc Natl Acad Sci U S A 98*, 4044-4049.

Six I, Gasan G, Mura E, Bordet R (2003). Beneficial effect of pharmacological mobilization of bone marrow in experimental cerebral ischemia. *Eur J Pharmacol 458*, 327-328.

Slevin M, Krupinski J, Slowik A, Kumar P, Szczudlik A, Gaffney J (2000). Serial measurement of vascular endothelial growth factor and transforming growth factor-beta1 in serum of patients with acute ischemic stroke. *Stroke 31*, 1863-1870.

Spera PA, Ellison JA, Feuerstein GZ, Barone FC (1998). IL-10 reduces rat brain injury following focal stroke. *Neurosci Lett 251*, 189-192.

Stoll G, Muller S, Schmidt B, van der Meide P, Jung S, Toyka KV, Hartung HP (1993). Localization of interferon-gamma and Ia-antigen in T cell line-mediated experimental autoimmune encephalomyelitis. *Am J Pathol. 142*, 1866-1875.

Stoll G, Jander S, Schroeter M (1998). Inflammation and glial responses in ischemic brain lesions. *Prog Neurobiol 56*, 49-71.

Stoll G, Jander S, Myers RR (2002). Degeneration and regeneration of the peripheral nervous system: from Augustus Waller's observations to neuroinflammation. *J Peripher Nerv Syst 7*, 13-27.

Stoll G, Schroeter M, Jander S, Siebert H, Wollrath A, Kleinschnitz C, Bruck W (2004). Lesion-associated expression of transforming growth factor-beta-2 in the rat nervous system: evidence for down-regulating the phagocytic activity of microglia and macrophages. *Brain Pathol 14*, 51-58.

Streit WJ (2002) Microglia as neuroprotective, immunocompetent cells of the CNS. *Glia 40*, 133-139.

Strijbos PJ, Rothwell NJ (1995). Interleukin-1 beta attenuates excitatory amino acid-induced neurodegeneration in vitro: involvement of nerve growth factor. *J Neurosci 15*, 3468-3474.

Stroemer RP, Rothwell NJ (1998). Exacerbation of ischemic brain damage by localized striatal injection of interleukin-1beta in the rat. *J Cereb Blood Flow Metab 18*, 833-839.

Takeda H, Spatz M, Ruetzler C, McCarron R, Becker K, Hallenbeck J (2002). Induction of mucosal tolerance to E-selectin prevents ischemic and hemorrhagic stroke in spontaneously hypertensive genetically stroke-prone rats. *Stroke 33*, 2156-2163.

Tasaki K, Ruetzler CA, Ohtsuki T, Martin D, Nawashiro H, Hallenbeck JM (1997). Lipopolysaccharide pre-treatment induces resistance against subsequent focal cerebral ischemic damage in spontaneously hypertensive rats. *Brain Res 74*, 267-270.

Tikka T, Fiebich BL, Goldsteins G, Keinanen R, Koistinaho J (2001) Minocycline, a tetracycline derivative, is neuroprotective against excitotoxicity by inhibiting activation and proliferation of microglia. *J Neurosci 21*, 2580-2588.

Touzani O, Boutin H, LeFeuvre R, Parker L, Miller A, Luheshi G, Rothwell N (2002). Interleukin-1 influences ischemic brain damage in the mouse independently of the interleukin-1 type I receptor. *J Neurosci 22*, 38-43.

Van Exel E, Gussekloo J, de Craen AJ, Bootsma-van der Wiel A, Frolich M, Westendorp RG (2002). Inflammation and stroke: the Leiden 85-Plus Study. *Stroke 33*, 1135-1138.

Veldhuis WB, Derksen JW, Floris S, Van Der Meide PH, De Vries HE, Schepers J, Vos IM, Dijkstra CD, Kappelle LJ, Nicolay K, Bar PR (2003). Interferon-beta blocks infiltration of inflammatory cells and reduces infarct volume after ischemic stroke in the rat. *J Cereb Blood Flow Metab 23*, 1029-1039.

Veltkamp R, Rajapakse N, Robins G, Puskar M, Shimizu K, Busija D (2002). Transient focal ischemia increases endothelial nitric oxide synthase in cerebral blood vessels. *Stroke 33*, 2704-2710.

Villa P, Bigini P, Mennini T, Agnello D, Laragione T, Cagnotto A, Viviani B, Marinovich M, Cerami A, Coleman TR, Brines M, Ghezzi P (2003). Erythropoietin selectively attenuates cytokine production and inflammation in cerebral ischemia by targeting neuronal apoptosis. *J Exp Med 198*, 971-975.

Vuorte J, Lindsberg PJ, Kaste M, Meri S, Jansson SE, Rothlein R, Repo H (1999). Anti-ICAM-1 monoclonal antibody R6.5 (Enlimomab) promotes activation of neutrophils in whole blood. *J Immunol 15*, 2353-2357.

Wallace MN, Bisland SK (1994). NADPH-diaphorase activity in activated astrocytes represents inducible nitric oxide synthase. *Neuroscience 59*, 905-919.

Wang X, Yue TL, Barone FC, White RF, Gagnon RC, Feuerstein GZ (1994). Concomitant cortical expression of TNF-alpha and IL-1 beta mRNAs follows early response gene expression in transient focal ischemia. *Mol Chem Neuropathol 23*, 103-114.

Wang X, Yue TL, White RF, Barone FC, Feuerstein GZ (1995a). Demonstration of increased endothelial-leukocyte adhesion molecule-1 mRNA expression in rat ischemic cortex. *Stroke 26*, 1665-1669.

Wang X, Yue TL, Barone FC, Feuerstein GZ (1995b). Monocyte chemoattractant protein-1 messenger RNA expression in rat ischemic cortex. *Stroke 26*, 661-665.

Wang X, Barone FC, Aiyar NV, Feuerstein GZ (1997). Interleukin-1 receptor and receptor antagonist gene expression after focal stroke in rats. *Stroke 28*, 155-161.

Wang X, Feuerstein GZ, Xu L, Wang H, Schumacher WA, Ogletree ML, Taub R, Duan JJ, Decicco CP, Liu RQ (2004). Inhibition of tumor necrosis factor-alpha-converting enzyme by a selective antagonist protects brain from focal ischemic injury in rats. *Mol Pharmacol 65*, 890-896.

Watson BD, Dietrich D, Busto R, Wachtel MS, Ginsberg MD (1985). Induction of reproducible brain infarction by photochemically initiated thrombosis. *Ann Neurol 17*, 497-504.

Weih M, Kallenberg K, Bergk A, Dirnagl U, Harms L, Wernecke KD, Einhaupl KM (1999). Attenuated stroke severity after prodromal TIA: a role for ischemic tolerance in the brain? *Stroke 30*, 1851-1854.

Weiner HL (1997). Oral tolerance: immune mechanisms and treatment of autoimmune diseases. *Immunol Today 18*, 335-343.

Weiner HL (2001). Oral tolerance: immune mechanisms and the generation of Th3-type TGF-beta secreting regulatory cells. *Microbes Infect 3*, 947-954.

Wekerle H, Linington C, Lassmann H, Meyermann R (1986). Cellular immune reactivity within the CNS. *Trends Neurosci 9*, 271-277.

Wheeler RD, Boutin H, Touzani O, Luheshi GN, Takeda K, Rothwell NJ (2003). No role for interleukin-18 in acute murine stroke induced brain injury. *J Cereb Blood Flow Metab 23*, 531-535.

Xu Y, Song G (2004) The role of CD40-CD154 interaction in cell immunoregulation. *J Biomed Sci 11*, 426-438.

Yamasaki Y, Matsuo Y, Matsuura N, Onodera H, Itoyama Y, Kogure K (1995). Transient increase of cytokine-induced neutrophil chemoattractant, a member of the interleukin-8 family, in ischemic brain areas after focal ischemia in rats. *Stroke 26*, 318-322.

Yamashita K, Vogel P, Fritze K, Back T, Hossmann KA, Wiessner C (1996). Monitoring the temporal and spatial activation pattern of astrocytes in focal cerebral ischemia using in situ hybridization to GFAP mRNA: comparison with sgp-2 and hsp70 mRNA and the effect of glutamate receptor antagonists. *Brain Res 735*, 285-297.

Yanamoto H, Hashimoto N, Nagata I, Kikuchi H (1998). Infarct tolerance against temporary focal ischemia following spreading depression in rat brain. *Brain Res 784*, 239-249.

Yilmaz G, Arumugam TV, Stokes KY, Granger DN (2006) Role of T lymphocytes and interferon-gamma in ischemic stroke. *Circulation 113*, 2105-2112.

Yoshida T, Limmroth V, Irikura K, Moskowitz MA (1994). The NOS inhibitor, 7-nitroindazole, decreases focal infarct volume but not the response to topical acetylcholine in pial vessels. *J Cereb Blood Flow Metab 14*, 924-929.

Yrjanheikki J, Tikka T, Keinanen R, Goldsteins G, Chan PH, Koistinaho J (1999). A tetracycline derivative, minocycline, reduces inflammation and protects against focal cerebral ischemia with a wide therapeutic window. *Proc Natl Acad Sci U S A 96*, 13496-13500.

Zaremba J, Losy J (2003). Interleukin-18 in acute ischaemic stroke patients. *Neurol Sci 24*, 117-124.

Zavala F, Abad S, Ezine S, Taupin V, Masson A, Bach JF (2002). G-CSF therapy of ongoing experimental allergic encephalomyelitis via chemokine- and cytokine-based immune deviation. *J Immunol 168*, 2011-2019.

Zhai QH, Futrell N, Chen FJ (1997). Gene expression of IL-10 in relationship to TNF-alpha, IL-1beta and IL-2 in the rat brain following middle cerebral artery occlusion. *J Neurol Sci 152*, 119-124.

Zhang F, Iadecola C (1993). Nitroprusside improves blood flow and reduces brain damage after focal ischemia. *Neuroreport 4*, 559-562.

Zhang F, Iadecola C (1994). Reduction of focal cerebral ischemic damage by delayed treatment with nitric oxide donors. *J Cereb Blood Flow Metab 14*, 574-580.

Zhang RL, Chopp M, Zalonga C, Jiang N, Gautam SC, Tang WX, Tsang W, Anderson DC, Manning AM (1995a). The temporal profiles of ICAM-1 protein and mRNA expression after transient MCAO occlusion in the rat. *Brain Res 682*, 182-188.

Zhang RL, Chopp M, Li Y, Zaloga C, Zhang ZG, Jiang N, Jones ML, Miyasaka M, Ward PA (1995b). Anti-ICAM-1 antibody reduces ischemic cell damage after transient but not permanent MCAO occlusion in the Wistar rat. *Stroke 26*, 1438-1443.

Zhang ZG, Chopp M, Powers C (1997). Temporal profile of microglial response following transient (2h) middle cerebral artery occlusion. *Brain Res 744*, 189-198.

In: Inflammation Research Perspectives
Editor: Giacomo T. Romano, pp. 113-168
ISBN: 978-1-60021-845-3

Chapter VI

BASIC CONCEPTS OF INFLAMMATION – FROM PIONEER STUDIES UNTIL NOW

Elzbieta Kolaczkowska, Magdalena Chadzinska and Barbara Plytycz
Department of Evolutionary Immunobiology, Institute of Zoology, Jagiellonian University, PL 30-060 Krakow, Poland.

ABSTRACT

The hallmarks of inflammation were described some 2000 years ago by Cornelius Celsus as "*rubor et tumor cum calore et dolore*" meaning "redness and swelling with heat and pain". In the 19th century this definition was extended by "*functio laesa*" (loss of function). This chapter provides the updated state of knowledge concerning major cellular and molecular mechanisms of this process, with a special emphasis on early events of acute inflammation: changes in a vascular permeability, formation of chemotactic gradient, and a local accumulation of inflammatory cells and molecules. The role of mast cells, macrophages and neutrophils is highlighted, and special attention is given to the soluble mediators of inflammation, such as histamine, kinins, acute phase proteins, lipid mediators, chemokines, metalloproteinases and proinflammatory cytokines, including anti-nociceptive endogenous opioids. Cytokines produced during inflammation act not only locally but also affect the central nervous system and induce changes called "sickness behaviour": depress animal mobility, exploration of physical and social environment, reduce food and water intake, and impair learning and memory.

In this chapter, participation of inflammation in the homeostatic system of the body is illustrated by the results obtained by our group during studies on peritoneal inflammation induced in representatives of mammals, amphibians, and fish. Experimental peritonitis is a very convenient model for the precise quantitative analysis of inflammatory cells and soluble factors that may be easily washed out from the inflamed peritoneal cavity of vertebrate animals. The course of inflammation depends on the kind and dose of stimulus applied, and on the investigated animals. Moreover, it may differ between animals matched according to strain, gender, and age due to some common laboratory practices such as handling, injections, or social stress such as isolation or grouping. In ectothermic vertebrates, the course of inflammation is modified by ambient temperature and season, which indicates its dependence on the annual endogenous rhythms of the body. Supplementation of inflammation-inducing agent with morphine abolishes pain, and reduces influx of leukocytes into peritoneal cavity as well as levels of plasma chemotactic factors in fish (salmon and goldfish) and several (but not all) strains of mice but in none of the investigated amphibian species. Time-dependent changes of cells and molecules in the focus of inflammation are accompanied by the pronounced changes of animal behaviour (pain symptoms) and levels of mediators (corticosteroids, endogenous opioids).

1. Defining Inflammation

Inflammation [Latin: *inflammatio*; *inflammare*; to set on fire] is a response of the body evoked by the destruction of its own tissues or by the invasion of foreign material and serves to destroy both the harmful agent and the injured tissue. Inflammation occurs in vascularized tissue and is aimed to deliver defensive materials (cells and fluid) to the site of injury/infection [1,2]. Inflammation consists of phases that follow each other no matter what its cause and localization. These are increased permeability of local blood vessels, directed migration of leukocytes (chemotaxis) to the inflammatory focus, elimination of pathogens/cause and termination of inflammation [1,3-7].

The inflammatory responses are commonly classified into two major categories: acute and chronic inflammation; and this division is based on the duration and on the involved cell types. However, such a classification is rather artificial as these processes are not independent and in fact overlap each other. Acute inflammation is short-term (minutes to days) but if its cause is not removed it can turn into chronic inflammation, which can persist for months, years or a lifetime [1]. Nevertheless, the acute inflammation is not always followed by chronic response and chronic reaction may start immediately after injury, following just a minor acute phase (e.g. in tuberculosis) [8].

Acute inflammation is characterized by neutrophil infiltration and edema, while the chronic process is manifested by subsequent predominance of macrophages and lymphocytes [1]. To some degree this also occurs during the normal healing process (e.g. macrophage infiltration) but becomes exaggerated and chronic when there is ineffective elimination of foreign materials. Moreover, chronic inflammation is often associated with fusion of mononuclear cells to form multinucleated giant cells, which eventually become *granuloma* [9]. Neutrophils and macrophages eliminate injurious agents by non-specific means (and therefore are called: innate immune responses) but lymphocytes specifically recognize foreign materials thereby initiating the sophisticated immune response (adaptive immunity) that involves immune memory (for review see [10]).

1.1. Understanding What Inflammation Is

The four cardinal signs of inflammation were described already by Celsus (30 B.C.-38 A.D.) as *calor* (heat), *rubor* (redness), *tumor* (swelling) and *dolor* (pain). These fundamental features were already known and recognized by ancient Egyptian, Mesopotamian, Greek, and Chinese physicians [11]; however, they were not explained in any scientific terms until 1867. Since then, the redness and heat are attributed to increased blood flow at the inflammatory site, the swelling to the exudation of cells and fluid, and the pain to the direct effects of mediators [12]. The "loss of function" (*functio laesa*) is claimed to be the fifth sign added by Galen to the four cardinal signs of Celsus.

The pioneering work on mechanisms involved in inflammation was provided by Elya Metchnikoff (1845-1916) whose studies of starfish larvae (*Bipinnaria*) and water flea (*Daphnia*) led to discovery of phagocytosis [13,14]. He showed that the basic feature of cells involved in inflammation is their capacity to phagocytose, i.e. to ingest target material to eliminate it. The observations conducted on invertebrates also indicated that this defense mechanism is phylogenetically conserved. The studies on phagocytosis together with those on humoral response (antibodies) by Paul Ehrlich (1854-1915) led to conclusion of the dual nature of inflammation, i.e. cellular and humoral (fluid) [1].

1.2. Experimental Models of Inflammation

Experimentally induced inflammation is an approach to study cellular and humoral mechanisms controlling this process, and representatives of different vertebrate groups have proven to be useful for those studies. The convenience of experimental models relies on a possibility of precise quantification of inflammation-related cells and soluble factors in samples collected from inflammatory focus.

The most common models of acute inflammation include:

- subcutaneous air pouch; s.c. injection of air followed by administration of inflammatory agent (e.g. [15-18]),
- paw edema; injection of irritant into the plantar surface of the hindpaw (e.g. [19-21]),
- sepsis, i.e. systemic inflammatory response; e.g. septic peritonitis can be induced by cecal ligation and puncture (e.g.[22,23]) or i.p./i.v. application of endotoxin (e.g.[24,25]),
- pleuritis and peritonitis; injection of irritant into pleural or peritoneal cavities, respectively (e.g. [3,4,15,26-30]).

The experimental models of inflammation differ not only by their location within the body but also by the inflammatory agent applied. The intention is not to list all of them here, so only some of the most representative will be named. The inflammatory agents used in animal models are either "true" pathogens (e.g *Escherichia coli* or *Staphylococcus aureus*) or their immuno-stimulatory components. The latter group includes the constituents of bacteria (e.g. lipopolysaccharide component of Gram-negative bacteria; LPS) and fungi (e.g. polysaccharide component of the cell walls of *Saccharomyces cerevisiae*; zymosan) that mimic the infection with respective pathogens as they contain the active antigens [31]. Also, non-pathogenic irritants are being used. For example, medium (e.g. sterile Thioglycollate broth [6,26,32-34]), plant extracts (e.g. colloid component of the cell wall of sea weeds, carrageenan) (e.g. [35]), clay (mineral; kaolin) (e.g. [36]), and dextran gel (sephadex) (e.g. [37,38]) can be used for induction of inflammation.

The inflammatory profile, i.e. quantity and quality of infiltrating cells and secreted mediators and their kinetics, depends on the nature (antigenicity) of applied irritant as well as on its structure, being either soluble (e.g. Thioglycollate, carrageenan) or particulate (LPS, zymosan, sephadex) [32,39,40].

Among the named experimental inflammatory models, peritonitis (peritoneal inflammation) represents a convenient model to study acute inflammation, as the peritoneum is a rich source of resident and inflammatory (upon proper stimulation) leukocytes, as well as inflammatory mediators, that are easy to retrieve and quantify [2]. In the present chapter some inflammatory phenomena will be illustrated by data obtained from studies on peritonitis induced by several types of irritants (e.g. zymosan and thioglycollate) in different groups of vertebrates.

2. Kinetics of Inflammation

Sequential events occurring in a course of inflammation follow the same general pattern disregard on its cause or localization in a body. Firstly, upon tissue injury or antigen penetration, vasodilatation and permeability of local blood vessels increases that is followed by leukocyte infiltration (by inflammatory neutrophils and macrophages) into the inflammatory focus (Figures 1-5). If elimination of antigens by the cells is successful a termination of inflammation takes place; otherwise it turns into chronic inflammation.

2.1. Vascular Permeability Changes

Increased vascular permeability is one of the primary steps initiating the inflammatory process (Figure 1), as it leads to the leakage of plasma into the inflammatory site and therefore is the key factor for the production of inflammatory exudate. Plasma, in turn, contains some first-line chemotactic factors mediating subsequent cellular extravasation to the inflamed tissue [2,6,7,41,42].

In normal blood vessels, the endothelium forms a continuous, semipermeable barrier [43]. In response to inflammatory stimuli, the endothelial barrier becomes less restrictive, resulting in increased water and protein permeability. Two mechanisms can account for this increase in permeability: paracellular (i.e., between endothelial cells) pathway and transcytotic (i.e. vesicular transport through endothelial cell) pathway [43]. Local release of vasomediator(s) causes the venular endothelia to develop openings or gaps (0.1-0.4 μm in diameter) between adjacent and contracted endothelial cells [44]. The mechanism leading to inter-endothelial cell gap formation and increased permeability to macromolecules is initiated by a rise in $[Ca^{2+}]_i$ but only in the absence of an increase in cAMP [45]. The latter phenomenon is due to the fact that endothelial cells express the Ca^{2+}-inhibited isoform of adenylyl cyclase, the enzyme responsible for cAMP synthesis. Moreover, the production of cAMP is regulated (both stimulatory and inhibitory) by ligand-receptor-G protein activation of adenylyl cyclases (Moore et al. 1998). Thus, direct $[Ca^{2+}]_i$ elevating agents (without activation of G proteins; unlike vasomediators) cannot increase microvascular permeability [43,46]. This serves as an important homeostatic mechanism controlling endothelial cell barrier function [47]. Inflammation may also increase the selected transport of macromolecules (e.g. albumins) through the cells. This transcellular pathway is mediated by a specific docking protein (gp60) but the whole molecular mechanism remains unclear [43,48].

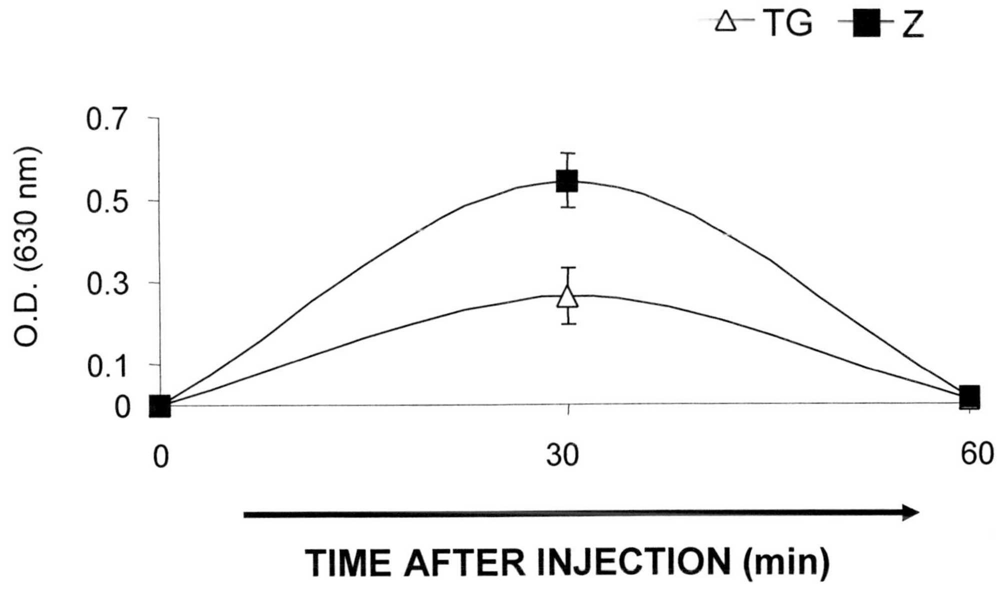

Figure 1. Changes in vascular permeability during experimental peritonitis induced by either zymosan (2mg/ml; 0.5 ml/mouse; Z) or 3% thioglycollate (TG) in male Swiss mice. Immediately after induction of inflammation mice were intravenously injected with Evans blue solutions (10mg/ml; 0.3ml/mouse) and their peritoneal cavity was lavaged with 1 ml of saline at the selected time points (time 0 - intact animals, 30min and 60min after irritant injection). Peritoneal fluid was centrifuged and absorbance of the dye (Evans blue binds covalently to plasma albumins) in the supernatant was measured with spectrophotometer at 650 nm. Means ± SE, n=4-8.

The increase in vascular permeability occurs within minutes and was first described by Majno & Palade [49] upon local injection of histamine and serotonin. Subsequently Majno et al. [50] showed that the increased permeability induced by histamine and serotonin was confined to the venules and did not involve the true capillaries. The same mechanism was demonstrated to operate for various mediators (for review see [51]).

The microvessels are not passive pipes through which exchange occurs but are in fact dynamic structures [52]. Under normal circumstances, high hydrostatic pressure forces fluid out of the vessels into the extravascular space, but the high colloid osmotic pressure inside the vessel (due to plasma proteins) favors fluid return to the vascular compartment. During inflammation, the capillary hydrostatic pressure is increased (due to dilated arterioles), and because there is a subsequent escape of plasma proteins into the extravascular space, the colloid osmotic pressure decreases. Consequently, much more fluid leaves the vessels than is returned to them [1].

The increase of vascular permeability can result from direct endothelial damage such as that produced by physical injury, otherwise it is due to action of low molecular weight chemical mediators that initiate inflammatory reactions [51,53].

2.2. Chemotaxis and Leukocyte Infiltration

Chemotaxis of leukocytes is a central event during inflammatory response, which acts to localize cells to the site of infection or injury (Figures 2, 3).

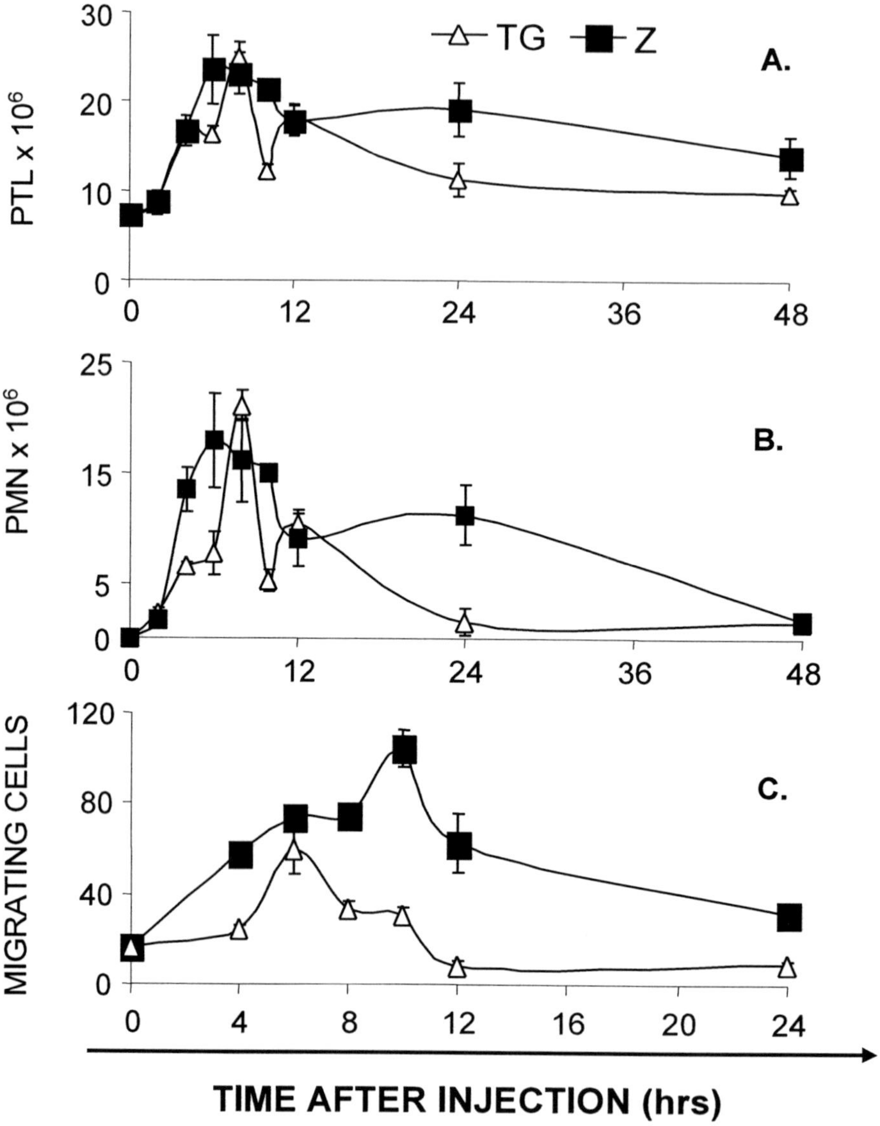

Figure 2. Kinetics of peritoneal inflammation in male Swiss mice. Animals were i.p. injected with either zymosan (2mg/ml; 0.5 ml/mouse; Z) or 3% thioglycollate (TG) and sacrificed at the selected time points after treatment; time 0 – intact animals. Peritoneal cavity was lavaged with 1 ml of saline and (A) the total number of peritoneal leukocytes (PTL) and among them (B) polymorphonuclear leukocytes (PMN) was counted with a hemocytometer following staining with Turk's solutions (0.01% crystal violet in 3% acetic acid). Total level of chemoattractants (C) in blood plasma was measured as the number of bone marrow cells from intact mice responding (migrating cells) to the tested plasma in a 48-well chemotactic chamber (for method see [33]. Means ± SE, n=4-8.

The efficient recruitment of leukocytes to the inflammatory focus depends on the sequential cascade of leukocyte-endothelial cell adhesive interactions [54,55]. This multistep process includes: *rolling* of leukocytes along the vessel wall, *adhesion* - tight binding of leukocytes to the endothelium, and migration of leukocytes through the endothelial junctions - *diapedesis* [56,57]. Various chemoattractants play a fundamental role in this process by attracting and stimulating specific subsets of leukocytes [58] (compare with a paragraph 4.5).

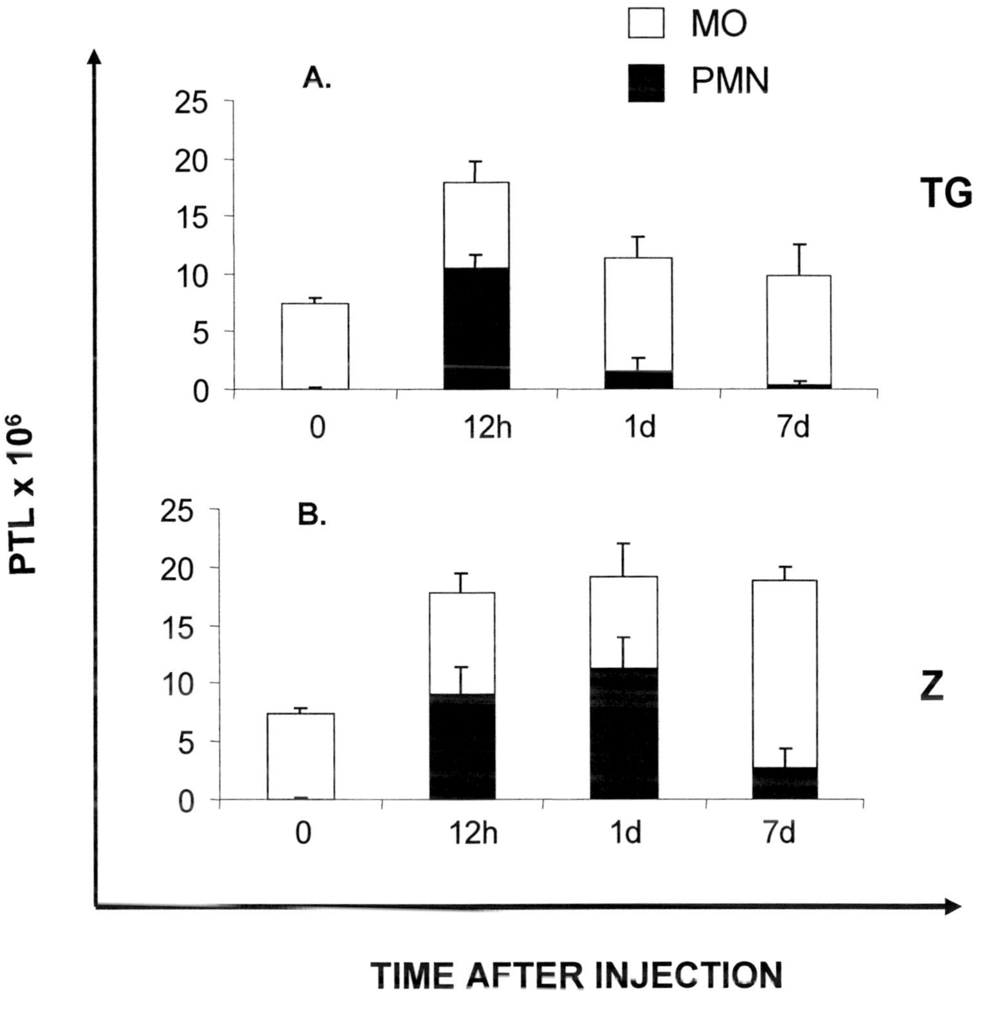

Figure 3. Changes in the number of mononuclear (MO) and polymorphonuclear (PMN) leukocytes retrieved from peritoneal cavity of the male Swiss mice. Animals were i.p. injected with either (A) 3% thioglycollate – TG or (B) zymosan – Z (2mg/ml; 0.5 ml/mouse) and sacrificed at the selected time points after treatment; time 0 – intact animals. Peritoneal cavity was lavaged with 1 ml of saline and total leukocyte (PTL) numbers were counted with a hemocytometer following staining with Turk's solutions (0.01% crystal violet in 3% acetic acid). Means ± SE, n=4-8.

The initial rolling of leukocytes results from a loose, transient adhesion mediated by three types of selectins, a family of adhesion molecules. L-selectins are constantly expressed on leukocytes whereas P- and E-selectins are expressed on stimulated endothelium. P-selectins are rapidly mobilized from intracellular stores by e.g. histamine, but E-selectins, inducible by e. g. IL-1, TNF or LPS, require *de novo* protein synthesis [59]. During this phase leukocytes sample the endothelium and if the specific chemoattractants are found they can be activated to become firmly adherent [60]. A tight adhesion is established by binding of integrins on white blood cells to the cell adhesion molecules on endothelium. Integrins, β_2 (CD11/CD18) and β_1 (VLA-4: very late antigen) expressed on leukocytes interact with intercellular adhesion molecule-1 (ICAM-1) and vascular cell adhesion molecule-1 (VCAM-1) on endothelium, respectively [61,62]. Firm adhesion is facilitated by two events: an increase in number of ICAM-1 and VCAM-1 molecules on endothelium induced by IL-1, TNF or LPS, and an increased affinity of integrins on leukocytes for their endothelial ligands [63]. During this phase on the endothelium, the leukocytes can be fully activated and their cytoskeleton undergoes an intense reorganization preparing the cells for diapedesis [54]. The emigration process is facilitated by leukocyte crawling toward and passing between the endothelial cells, and involves binding between platelet-endothelial cell adhesion molecule-1 (PECAM-1) on leukocytes and endothelium [64,65]. The leukocyte passage takes place at tricellular corners between the endothelial cells [66]. Subsequently leukocytes migrate through the underlining tissues and are guided to the inflammatory focus by increasing chemotactic gradients [63]. Lymphocyte extravasation from the blood occurs via high endothelial venules (HEVs) that are specialized post-capillary venules found in lymphoid tissues [67,68].

More recently, an alternative pathway was described in which α_4-integrins mediate both, the rolling and adhesion steps, in chronically inflamed postcapillary venules [69,70].

2.2.1. Metalloproteinases

Upon receiving a chemotactic signal leukocytes start to extravasate but after passing through the endothelial junctions in a process of diapedesis they must face a problem of degrading basement membrane; and after successful extravasation they must be able to migrate through the extracellular matrix following chemotactic gradient

Leukocytes can achieve those actions by releasing degradative enzymes into the pericellular space [71]. Among the proteolytic enzymes, Zn^{2+}-endopeptidases of matrix metalloproteinase (MMP) family carry an activity that can trigger break down of vascular basement membrane and degradation of extracellular matrix macromolecules (ECM) [72]. The MMPs, which can cleave most of the constituents of the ECM, are secreted in a latent form of pro-enzymes and thus require activation by the cysteine switch mechanism i.e. removal of the cysteine sulfhydryl group in the pro-domain [73-75]. Among MMPs, gelatinases that belong to the secreted members constitute a terminal step in the enzyme cascade that processes the ECM, including basement membranes as their substrates include types IV and V collagen, fibronectin, elastin, and denaturated interstitial collagen (gelatin) [76-78]. In particular two members are distinguished in this group, MMP-2 (65-75 kDa; gelatinase A) and MMP-9 (>85-kDa; gelatinase B) with the former being constitutively present in all body fluids and the latter being inducible [73,74]. Gelatinase B proenzyme can be activated by components of the plasminogen system [77-80] but the activation is achieved mainly by a protease network [79]. Role of MMP-9 in neutrophil recrutment into the inflammatory focus was shown by numerous studies [e.g. 81-82]. Moreover, also metalloelastase (MMP-12) and neutrophil elastase were shown to be crucial for penetratation of basement membrane by leukocytes, both *in vitro* and *in vivo* [83-85]. An important mechanism for the regulation of the activity of MMPs is via binding to a family of homologous secreted proteins referred to as the tissue inhibitors of metalloproteinases (TIMP-1 to TIMP-4) [86]; and in the circulation any MMP activity can be inhibited by the broad-spectrum protease inhibitor α_2-macroglobulin [87,88]. The TIMPs inhibit metalloproteinases rather selectively and reversibly, in a 1:1 stoichiometric manner [89]. Imbalance between MMPs and TIMPs activities has been observed in numerous pathological disorders, including asthma [90,91], atherosclerosis [91,92], inflammation [93,94], tumor growth and metastasis [94-96].

2.3. Elimination of Antigen

The major effector function of professional phagocytes, neutrophils and macrophages is to eliminate/kill infectious microorganisms. Thus, upon initiation of phagocytosis, two microbicidal mechanisms are concomitantly activated: the oxygen-dependent ("oxidative burst") and oxygen-independent (enzymatic) cytotoxic processes that occur mainly within phagolysosomes [97].

Oxidative burst, so called due to the 50- to 100-fold increase in oxygen consumption, leads to the production of reactive oxygen intermediates (ROI) and reactive nitrogen intermediates (RNI). The enzyme responsible for the increased oxygen uptake, NADPH oxidase, is inactive in dormant cells but upon activation it mediates the formation of superoxide (O_2^-) as it catalyses the reduction of molecular oxygen by single electrons that originate from NADPH [98]. Most of the O_2^- reacts with itself that leads to formation of hydrogen peroxide (H_2O_2), which either occurs spontaneously or is catalyzed by superoxide dismutase (SOD) [99]. At the same time glucose is metabolized via hexose monophosphate (HMP) shunt in order to regenerate NADPH [1]. Neither superoxide (O_2^-) nor hydrogen peroxide (H_2O_2) contribute significantly to the killing but their formation is necessary for generation of other potent ROI, namely oxidizing radicals and oxidizing halogens [100]. Hydroxyl radical (OH•), the prototype of the oxidizing radicals, is formed by the Fe^{2+}-catalyzed decomposition of H_2O_2; and hypochlorous acid or hypochlorite (HOCl), the prototype of the oxidizing halogens, is generated by the reaction of H_2O_2 with the abundant Cl^- ions taken up from extracellular fluid. The reaction depends on presence of myeloperoxidase (MPO), an enzyme exclusively present in neutrophilic granules. However, during phagocytosis of a pathogen, neutrophils degranulate and release MPO into the extracellular enviroment from where it can be utilized by macrophages that bind the enzyme via their mannose receptors [101,102]. Next, the short-lived hypochlorous acid reacts with free amino acids (e.g. taurine, the most abundant amino acid in leukocytes) to form chlorinated amines (chloramines), e.g. long-lived taurine chloramine (TauCl) [103-105]. Hypochlorous acid can also react with hydrogen peroxide leading to formation of singlet oxygen ($^1O_2$).

The other oxygen-dependent mechanisms lead to production of reactive nitrogen intermediates (RNI), e.g. nitric oxide. Short-lived nitric oxide ($NO^{\bullet}$) is derived from the guanidino nitrogen in the conversion of L-arginine to L-citrulline and is subsequently converted into endporoducts, nitrite and nitrate [106,107]. The reaction is catalyzed by NO synthase (NOS) that exists in two isoforms, constitutive (cNOS) and inducible (iNOS), which is induced, for example, during inflammation [108].

The mechanisms by which different oxidants contribute to bacterial killing are still subject to investigation but in general, oxidants might arrest bacterial growth by inhibition of DNA synthesis or disruption of metabolic processes [109]. As lipids are their primary targets the cell membranes are especially at risk but they can also act on proteins and carbohydrates [99].

Apart from the oxidative killing pathway, the oxygen-independent mechanisms are also triggered upon phagocytosis as hydrolytic enzymes and antimicrobial polypeptides contained in cell granules are released into phagolysosomes. For example, proteases such as elastase and cathepsin G hydrolyze proteins in bacterial cell envelopes while lysozyme degrades the polysaccharide components [110,111]. Bactericidal/permeability-increasing protein (BPI) is highly toxic to gram-negative bacteria and can also neutralize the lipopolysaccharide component of their cell wall [112]. Lactoferrin sequesters free iron, thus preventing the growth of ingested microorganisms that survive the killing process [113]. Finally, defensins (small proteins) as well as complement components are lytic to broad range of bacteria, fungi, and some viruses [114,115]. The oxidative and non-oxidative processes can kill some microbes independently but their combination facilitates or increases substantially the killing potential, e.g. gram-negative bacteria are resistant to lysozyme unless they are subjected simultaneously to oxidants and/or complement factors, and lactoferrin increases bacterial permeability to lysozyme [116].

The killing processes are also potentially dangerous for the host tissue. Thus phagocytes contain endogenous antioxidants (e.g. vitamin C) that are in the reduced state during phagocytosis and therefore prevent death from oxidative suicide [117].

2.4. Termination of Inflammation

Inflammation persists (and becomes chronic) if the infectious agent is not removed but in most cases inflammation is the self-limiting process as several mediators contribute to its down-regulation [118-120].

For example, neutrophil-derived protein lipocortin 1 (LC1; annexin I) acts as a suppressor of eicosanoid production (via inhibition of PLA_2) and an autocrine mediator with an inhibitory action on diapedesis [121-123]. Externalization of LC1 on the plasma membrane of adherent neutrophils reduces their rate of passage through the endothelial gaps [124]. Lipocortin 1 expression is inducible by glucocorticoid hormones that are produced in adrenal glands in response to injury or infectious agents. Their mechanism of action includes both the suppression of pro-inflammatory mediators and the upregulation of at least one anti-inflammatory protein, LC1 [125].

The expression of anti-inflammatory cytokines occurs as a result of "negative feedback regulatory loop" as pro-inflammatory cytokines, produced in response to immune stimuli, in turn induce the synthesis of other cytokines, which have the ability to suppress their iducer [118,126]. Anti-inflammatory cytokines include interleukin-10 (IL-10), IL-4, IL-13, and transforming growth factor (TGF-β), as they suppress gene expression and synthesis of pro-inflammatory TNF-α, IL-1β and IL-6 [119,127]. Moreover, IL-10 inhibits production of oxygen and nitrogen intermediates by macrophages [128], downregulates cell membrane TNF receptors [129] and, together with IL-4, IL-13 and TGF-β, enhances synthesis of interleukin-1 receptor antagonist (IL-1Ra) [130]. IL-1Ra is a unique naturally occurring specific inhibitor that binds to the IL-1RI receptor but fails to bring about the subsequent interaction with AcP, thus does not signal and also by blocking the receptor prevents the action of IL-1α and IL-1β [119,131]. Recently, a novel interleukin-18 binding protein was described (IL-18BP) that neutralises IL-18 and was shown to share many characteristics with soluble IL-1 receptors [132]. Soluble receptors of IL-1 and TNF-α (sIL-1R and sTNFR) are other suppressory molecules that compete for specific cytokines with membrane-bound forms and modulate their action by acting as cytokine scavengers, cytokine carrier proteins and stabilizers (sTNFR), competitive cytokine inhibitors or antagonists [133,134]. In contrast, sIL-6R is able to form biologically active complexes with IL-6 [135,136] [137].

Also, the action of chemokines, considered pro-inflammatory mediators, is limited by suppressory mechanisms. They include 1) downregulation of the chemokine expression by anti-inflammatory cytokines IL-4 and IL-10 [127,138,139] 2) neutralization of chemokine activity by polyclonal autoantibodies, e.g. anti-IL-8 and anti-MCP-1 [140] 3) scavenging of free chemokines by cell surface receptors, e.g. on erythrocytes [141] and, 4) inhibition of responses to chemokines by chemokines themselves [142].

Once inflammation is terminated the tissue repair (i.e. wound healing) process takes place that closes the gaps and seals them with scar(s) [5].

3. Cells Participating in Inflammation

Critical role in orchestrating the inflammatory response is played by leukocytes and some other cells localized in the inflammatory locus. In a course of acute inflammation a major role is played by resident mast cells and tissue macrophages; and then infiltrating neutrophils and monocytes/macrophages.

3.1. Mast Cells

Mast cells [German: *mastzellen*; well-fed cells] contain numerous granules inside their cytoplasm [143]. The granules are the sites of storage of numerous mediators of which some can be constantly produced and then stored or alternatively produced *de novo* upon mast cell activation [144].

Mast cells reside at specific sites, frequently located strategically in tissues that are in contact with the external environment, and in nearness to blood or lymphatic vessels and to nerves [145,146]. This distribution places mast cells near pathogens that come in contact with the skin or mucosal surfaces and facilitates their exposure to blood-borne antigens. In turn, the mast cell distribution makes its products available to other cells of the connective tissue, epithelial cells, nerves and vascular endothelium [143,145].

In their granules mast cells carry numerous proteins and enzymes that include biogenic amines (histamine and, serotonin - in rodents), neutral proteases (chymease, tryptase, carboxypeptidase) and proteoglycans (heparin, chondroitin sulfate) [143,147-149] as well as inflammatory mediators. Upon activation (e.g. by inflammatory stimulus), mast cells release the prestored content of their granules and start to synthesize the other factors. In both cases similar groups of mediators are produced (cytokines, chemokines, growth factors) albeit particular members of each groups can differ [146,149-151]. For example, IL-8 can be stored in mast cell granules while MIP-1α, -1β and MCP-1 are produced upon activation [143,149,150].

Histamine is one of the most powerful mediators carried in mast cell granules (it occupies up to 10% of the granule content). Positively charged histamine and some other molecules (proteolytic enzymes, chemotactic factors, and serotonin in rodents) are noncovalently bound to negatively charged heparin (sulfated glycosaminoglycan) [152]. The latter feature counts for granules' staining with basic dyes and is common for mast cells and basophils. In fact these two types of cells are structurally and functionally related to each other although they originate from different precursors, and basophils, unlike mast cells, do not leave the circulation [150,153].

Mast cells express surface FcεRI receptors that bind with high affinity to the Fc portion of IgE antibody [154]. Recognition of a specific multivalent antigen by IgE antibodies bound to the cell receptors leads to the mast cell degranulation, i.e. they release the content of their granules [155]. Cross-linking of FcγRIII molecules also activates mast cells but the nature of released mediators may differ [156]. However, mast cells can also be stimulated by IgE-independent means as they can be activated by direct contact with infectious agents or with secreted microbial products, such as toxins and cell wall constituents e.g. lipopolysaccharide (LPS) and polysaccharide component of *Saccharomyces cerevisiae* (zymosan) [157-159]. Moreover, some host-derived factors generated during inflammation may cause mast cell activation, including complement-derived anaphylatoxins (C3a, C5a) [160], subfragments of fibrinogen and fibronectin [161], and β-chemokines (MIP-1α and MCP-1) [162].

Mast cells contribute to at least three main steps of inflammatory response. They increase vascular permeability via action of histamine, serotonin, leukotriene C_4 (LTC_4), and platelet activating factor (PAF), and contribute to cell recruitment and chemotaxis to the inflammatory site [2,5,6,163]. Chemokines (IL-8, MIP-1α, β and MCP-1) and LTB_4 recruit neutrophils and monocytes, and TNF-α increases expression of adhesion molecules (E-selectin, ICAM, VCAM) on endothelial cells [28,164,165] and thus promote cell migration to the inflammatory focus. Finally, released proteases cause a direct killing of infectious agents [146]. Recently, mast cells were also demonstrated to participate in antigen presentation to T lymphocytes via MHC II molecules [165,166], and their involvement in phagocytosis has been analyzed in detail [167,168].

Mast cell precursors originate from multipotencial haemopoietic stem cells (CFU-S), $CD34^+$ c-kit^+ $CD13^+$ cells in humans and Thy-1^{lo} c-kit^{hi} cells in mice, in the bone marrow

[169,170]. They then migrate in the blood stream and enter the tissues where they are able to differentiate into morphologically identifiable mast cells [171,172], and a common precursor can give rise to both CTMCs and MMCs [173]. Mast cells are heterogeneous and in rodents can be divided into two phenotypically distinct populations, namely connective tissue mast cells (CTMC) and mucosal mast cells (MMC) [174]. The CTMC can be distinguished from the MMC by their anatomical location, morphology and histochemical staining properties. The CTMC are present in the skin, peritoneal cavity and muscularis propia of the stomach. They contain many granules with large amounts of histamine and heparin [174] but produce very little leukotriene [175]. In contrast, the MMC store chondroitin sulfate E instead of heparin and relatively small quantities of histamine [174,176] but synthesize large amounts of leukotrienes [177]. In humans the mast cell heterogeneity is less apparent as the two mast cell types, MC_{TC} and MC_T, differ mainly by their granule content of neutral proteases: MC_{TC} contain both tryptase and chymase and MC_T tryptase only; they are found mainly in the skin and lung, respectively [147]. Moreover, mast cell populations can undergo significant changes in numbers and phenotype during immune or inflammatory responses, due to microenvironmental alterations in e.g. expression of major mast cell growth factors, stem cell factor (SCF) and IL-3 [150,178].

3.2. Macrophages

The monocyte and macrophage represent a circulating and a tissue phase of the same cell type. The cells derive from a common precursor in the bone marrow, and subsequently circulate as mature monocytes, then leave the bloodstream to enter peripheral tissues where they settle as macrophages (Mø) [179]. The tissue resident macrophages are present in multiple locations, including peritoneum (peritoneal Mø), lungs (alveolar Mø), liver (Kupffer cells), central nervous system (microglia), and lymph nodes (sinus histiocytes) [180]. This wide distribution makes the resident Mø well suited to provide an immediate defense against foreign elements prior to leukocyte migration [181]. Moreover, macrophages from different tissues exhibit a wide range of phenotypes with regards to both their morphology and function, due to the local environment, which gives them flexibility to respond to challenge [182].

Recently, a novel B-1/macrophage cell population was described, representing biphenotypic leukocytes of unique function that simultaneously express B lymphocyte (e.g. surface immunoglobulins) and macrophage (e.g. phagocytosis) characteristics [183, 184]. The B-1/macrophage cells can be generated from purified mouse B lymphocytes incubated in fibroblast-conditioned medium but they were also detected *in vivo* in mouse peritoneum [185]. Plytycz and Seljelid [186] hypothesized that B-1/Mø might represent 'living fossils' – evolving transition cells combining lymphocyte-derived specificity with the most ancient defense mechanism - phagocytosis.

Monocytes and macrophages belong to the Mononuclear Phagocyte System (MPS) and the wider Reticuloendothelial System (RES). The first represents mononuclear phagocytic cells (monocytes, Mø, and their precursors) while RES includes all specialized scavenger cells that actively engulf and process waste macromolecules and cells [187-189].

The Mø's ability to phagocytose was discovered already by Metchnikoff and represents one of the prominent, defining features of macrophages, thereby called, along with neutrophils, professional phagocytes [190]. The initial step in the phagocytosis involves recognition of a target by specific receptors, such as the mannose receptor (MR), that recognize conserved motifs on pathogens e.g. mannosylated motifs of zymosan [191]. The scavenger receptors of a class A (SR-A), including recently identified macrophage receptor with collagenous structure (MARCO), bind to microbial polyanions e.g. LPS [192,193]. Pathogens are also phagocytosed by complement receptors (CR) after relatively nonspecific opsonization with complement (C3b) and by Fc receptors after specific opsonization with antibodies (FcR) [194]. All these receptors induce rearrangements in the actin cytoskeleton that lead to the internalization of the particle; however, they operate via different molecular mechanisms [195].

Phagocytosis proceeds by the so-called "zipper" mechanism as macrophage plasma membrane actively encloses the particle in a vacuole, which later becomes a phagolysosome [196]. The Mø killing mechanisms involve the respiratory burst and nonoxidative, enzymatic antibacterial processes (compare with a paragraph 2.3). Macrophage subpopoulations might show heterogeneity in both phagocytic activity and generation of reactive oxygen species [197]. The oxygen-independent pathway involves lysozyme, lactoferrin, acid hydrolases, and defensins [198]. Moreover, it was recently reported that the Toll-like receptors sample the contents of the vacuole and trigger an inflammatory response appropriate to defence against the specific organism [199].

Apart from scavenger role in the clearance of non-self materials (i.e. infectious agents), macrophages also phagocytose altered-self materials e.g. senescent red blood cells, immune complexes, inflammatory products, and apoptotic cells [182,200].

Resident resting tissue macrophages are usually relatively inactive immunologically, having low oxygen consumption, low levels of MHC II, and little or no cytokine secretion; however, they are phagocytic and chemotactic and retain some proliferative capacity [181]. Hamilton and Adams [201] defined two stages of macrophage activation as "primed" and "fully activated". In the "primed" state Mø exhibit enhanced MHC II expression, antigen presentation, and oxygen consumption but reduced proliferative capacity. The agents that prime Mø for activation are operationally termed macrophage-activating factor(s) (MAF) and include interferon γ (IFN-γ) of T lymphocyte-origin, and TNF-α [181]. Primed Mø respond to secondary stimuli to become "fully activated", a state defined by inability to proliferate, high oxygen consumption, killing of infectious agents, and maximal secretion of pro-inflammatory cytokines, lipid mediators, reactive oxygen products and nitric oxide [201]. Agents capable of providing secondary signals are diverse and frequently supplied by microbial or fungal cell wall products, i.e. LPS and zymosan, respectively [202]. The first signal lowers the dose recruitment for the second thus the causative agents can work co-operatively, although they might also work independently [201].

During inflammation the resident macrophages are among first cells to respond as they actively phagocytise the infectious agents and release vasoactive and chemotactic factors. The first exudatory cells to arrive to the inflammatory focus are neutrophils (Figures 2B, 3), which are followed by inflammatory macrophages in a second wave (Figure 3) [1]. Circulating monocytes provide a mobile source of functionally competent immunocytes capable of infiltrating the tissues where they become macrophages [181]. Therefore both resident and exudatory Mø are essential in the course of inflammatory response, with the latter type especially involved in chronic inflammation.

Apart from involvement in nonspecific immunity, macrophages participate in adaptive immunity via their ability to process and present antigens to T lymphocytes, in the context of MHC (major histocompatibility complex) class II, and to produce lymphocyte-activating cytokines. In turn, activated lymphocytes may modulate Mø action through cellular interactions and soluble products [200,203]. However, monocytes/macrophages that phagocytosed bacteria reveal reduced expression of HLA class II (designation for human MHC) and some intercellular adhesion molecules [204] as well as impaired antigen presentation [205]. Moreover, the phagocytosis of bacteria by monocytes/Mø was demonstrated to induce their apoptosis (programmed cell death) as evidenced by DNA fragmentation into oligosomes ("DNA ladder") that is a distinguished feature of apoptosis [206]. On the other hand, however, pro-inflammatory cytokines, including TNF-α, IL-1β and GM-CSF, prevent monocyte spontaneous apoptosis [207].

The capacity to phagocytose is a fundamental undisputed property of macrophages; nevertheless, it cannot obscure the other properties of these cells [179]. Macrophages are in fact multifunctional cells as they participate in specific immunity by antigen presentation (see above), and produce and release more than one hundred potent mediators (for review see [196,198]).

3.3. Neutrophils

Neutrophils (polymorphonuclear leukocytes) consist 50 to 60% of the total circulating leukocytes and constitute the "first line of defense" against infectious agents or "non-self" substances that penetrate the body, as they are the first cells to be recruited to the sites of infection in a response to chemotactic factors [208] (Figures 2, 3). They mature in the bone marrow before being released into the circulation where they spend only 6 to 10 hours prior to marginating and entering intravascular marginated pools where they survive for 1 to 2 days, without ability to multiply [209]. Thus the presence of neutrophils in the tissues indicates ongoing infection, as they do not leave the blood otherwise. At the inflammatory focus they bind to opsonized infectious agents and infected cells via antibody (Fc) and/or complement (C3b) receptors initiating the phagocytic process [210]. During phagocytosis, cytosolic granules fuse with the invaginating plasma membrane to form a phagolysosome into which they release their contents [211]. There are four types of neutrophil granules which contain, for example, lysozyme proteases, defensins, myeloperoxidase (MPO), and antimicrobial pepetides (lysozyme, lactofferin, bactericidal/permeability-inducing protein) [212]. Neutrophilic killing mechanisms consist of a combination of oxidative and enzymatic (oxygen-independent) processes that are activated simultaneously upon initiation of phagocytosis [213] (compare with a paragraph 2.3). Spent neutrophils undergo apoptosis at the inflammatory site, and are subsequently phagocitized by macrophages [214,215]. This stops disintegration *in vivo*, which would otherwise expel neutrophilic cytotoxic content into the extracellular milieu [216]. Interestingly, the phagocytosis of bacteria slows down the spontaneously occuring apoptosis of neutrophils [206]. Also the inflammatory mediators (e.g. GM-CSF, TNF-α, LTB4) prolong the functional life span of neutrophils through inhibition of apoptosis [217]. This might represent a mechanism prolonging survival of neutrophils engaged in phagocytosis, in order to avoid unnecessary involvement of specific immune response [206].

Neutrophils were also demonstrated to synthesize and secrete some cytokines including IL-1β, IL-6, and TNF-α [218] as well as some chemotactic factors. The latter group includes IL-8, macrophage inflammatory protein α and β (MIP-1α, β) and monocyte chemoattractant protein (MCP-1) [219-221]. These data origin mainly from *in vitro* studies and they were also confirmed in some experimental *in vivo* models [28,222,223]. The neutrophilic origin of pro-inflammatory cytokines would explain their early appearance during inflammation, even before macrophage influx, and the fact that PMN produce IL-8, a major chemoattractant for neutrophils, suggest that once they arrive at the inflammatory site, they can promote the further recruitment of neutrophils [224]. On the other hand, MIP-1α, MIP-1β, and MCP-1 are chemoattractants for monocytes/macrophages and are therefore responsible for their subsequent accumulation [220].

Moreover, neutrophils are potent producers of lipid mediators which can modulate both the inflammatory response and neutrophil function [225]. Among them, leukotriene B_4 is a strong neutrophil chemoattractant while platelet-activating factor (PAF) directly primes superoxide generation and enzyme release. However, prostaglandins suppress most neutrophil functions [226,227].

Recently it was suggested that neutrophils might also provide an additional, missing link between innate and acquired immunity via generation of reactive chloramines (for review see [228]). Neutrophils cooperate with Mø and other professional antigen presenting cells (APC), enhancing uptake and proteolysis of antigens by their chlorination. The phagocytosis, however, occurs without triggering inflammatory mediators such as TNF-α, NO and prostaglandins [104]. Since many of these products are inhibitory for T cells, this activity will also indirectly potentiate the specific T-cell-mediated response [104,228].

4. Inflammatory Mediators

Inflammatory leukocytes are able to achieve most of their functions through a release of certain factors described commonly as inflammatory mediators. Nevertheless, the mediators can also be produced by cells other then leukocytes and their functions extend beyond the immunological system.

4.1. Histamine

The vasoactive mediators were believed to act sequentially in the course of an acute inflammatory reaction [229] but there is no evidence that this actually occurs [230]. An exception is histamine, which in fact is released as the first mediator. Histamine (β-imidazolyethylamine) is stored preformed in the cytoplasmic granules of mast cells and thereby is immediately available [231,232]. However, not all tissue histamine is associated with mast cells, and depending upon the species, histamine has been detected in basophils [233], platelets [234], endothelial cells [235,236], and neurons [237]. In addition, there is evidence that histamine synthesis can be induced, and histamine made available in an unstored diffusable form, in tissues undergoing rapid tissue growth or repair [238,239]. These non-mast cell-associated sites of histamine production and storage indicate that histamine plays an important role not only in pathological but also in physiological processes.

In rodents, serotonin (5-hydroxytryptamine, 5-HT) is also carried by mast cells and therefore immediately released; otherwise it is contained in platelets [240]. Both vasoactive amines (histamine and serotonin) act in a similar manner causing contraction of smooth muscle (vasoconstriction), arteriolar dilatation (vasodilatation), and venular leakage (increased vascular permeability) [241].

Histamine is produced from histidine by histidine decarboxylase (HDC) [242] and its action is mediated by binding to specific cell-surface receptors [239]. The histamine receptors are widely distributed and also present on leukocytes [243]. The latter location indicates that apart from its early direct effects on inflammatory process, histamine can also modulate the immune response [244]. It was shown that histamine can activate NK cells [245], inhibit neutrophil chemotaxis and enzyme release [246], and suppress production of cytokines, including IL-2, IFN-γ, IL-1 [247] and TNF-α [248]. Moreover, histamine can inhibit a variety of lymphocyte functions, including proliferative response to mitogens [249], antibody synthesis by B cells [250], and cell-mediated cytolysis [251].

Histamine receptors can be divided into three types of extracellular receptors: H_1, H_2, and H_3 (for review see [252,253]). Moreover, the existence of a specific intracellular histamine receptor H_{IC} has been postulated but not proved to date [252,254]. The extracellular receptors belong to family of G-protein-coupled receptors and thereby comprise seven transmembrane (TM) domains and possess N-terminal glycosylation sites [252-254]). The third (TM3) and the fifth (TM5) transmembrane domains are responsible for binding of histamine [255].

4.2. Kinins

Kinins are very potent albeit short-lived (half-life of less than one minute) vasoactive peptides carried in blood in an inactive form as kininogens [256]. The kinin generation is initiated by activated Hageman factor of the clotting system, which activates prekallikrein, resulting in the production of kallikrein. Subsequently the kallikrein (specific protease) triggers kinin production, including the formation of bradykinin; however, alternative ways of activation are possible [256]. The action of kinins resembles that of histamine as they increase vascular permeability, cause vasodilation, and induce pain [1,257].

Most vasoactive peptides are produced and released locally by nerve cells and nerve terminals [258]. Among them, Substance P (released by endings of sensory C fibers) is especially relevant to inflammation as it functionally resembles bradykinin [259].

4.3. Acute Phase and Heat Shock Proteins

The acute phase proteins mediate the so-called acute phase response that is triggered by pro-inflammatory cytokines (TNF-α, IL-1β, IL-6) within hours of injury [1,260]. It manifests itself by drastically altered protein synthesis in liver as shown by the composition of the plasma: for some proteins, such as albumin, liver synthesis is decreased ("negative" acute phase proteins); for others, such as complement factor C3, alpha2-macroglobulin (α_2M) and fibrinogen, it is increased [260]. The major "positive" acute phase proteins, however, are serum amyloid A (SAA) and C-reactive protein (CRP), respectively [261,262]. The function of CRP is similar to that of IgG as it activates complement, binds Fc receptors and acts as an opsonin for various pathogens. However, unlike IgG, which specifically recognizes antigenic epitopes, CRP recognizes altered self and foreign molecules based on pattern recognition [263]. New findings suggest also an anti-inflammatory role for CRP because it modulates endotoxin shock and inhibits chemotaxis and the respiratory burst of neutrophils (for review see [262]).

The *in vivo* concentration of serum amyloid A (SAA) increases during inflammation by as much as 1000-fold yet its precise role in host defense has not been defined. The SAA is associated with high-density lipoproteins (HDL) and is potentially involved in the pathogenesis of several chronic inflammatory diseases [264]. It is the precursor of the amyloid A protein that is deposited in amyloid A amyloidosis, and it has also been implicated in the pathogenesis of atheroscelerosis and rheumatoid arthritis [261]. However, the presence of SAA was also detected in histologically normal tissues, suggesting its role as an "housekeeping" molecule (for review see [265]). The shut-off mechanism limiting the acute phase response involves mainly hypothalamic-pituitary-adrenal (HPA) axis, as TNF-α, IL-1 and IL-6 activate HPA leading to release of anti-inflammatory glucocorticoids [266].

The heat shock response is one of the most universal reactions known, which cells utilize to preserve cellular function and homeostasis, and heat shock proteins (HSPs) are among the most conserved molecules in phylogeny [267]. In fact they were detected in every species in which they have been sought (for review see [268]. Originally, HSPs were detected in *Drosophila* confronted with a sudden increase in temperature [269]. However, in mammalian cells, HSP synthesis can be also triggered by other stressful conditions such as cellular energy depletion (e.g. glucose deprivation), extreme concentrations of ions, heavy metals, and by oxygen radicals and inflammatory cytokines [270]. The heat shock proteins are divided into different families, according to molecular size [267]. Recently, interactions between the heat shock response and the nuclear factor-kappa B signaling pathway has been suggested [271].

In general the heat shock response serves as a defense mechanism against any kind of shock but more recently it has been found that several heat shock proteins play a more general role as house-keeping proteins [268]. The mechanism by which the heat shock response protects against inflammation-induced injury is not clear but it may involve the ability of HSPs to inhibit pro-inflammatory mediators [272]. The heat shock response has been demonstrated to inhibit expression of TNF-α, IL-1β, RANTES, and cytokine-mediated expression of inducible nitric oxide synthase (iNOS) [273]. The above inhibition might be, however, a consequence of heat shock response-induced inhibition of nuclear factor-kappaB

(NF-κB), a transcription factor involved in the regulation of many pro-inflammatory mediators [274].

4.4. Lipid Mediators

The lipid mediators consist of derivatives of arachidonic acid: eicosanoids and platelet activating factors (PAFs) [275]. The collective name of eicosanoids is used to describe a range of widely differing chemical substances (leukotrienes, hydroxy acids, prostanoids: prostaglandins and thromboxanes) that are produced by cells from polyunsaturated fatty acids, particularly arachidonic acid, and which contain a 20-carbon (C_{20}) atom chain [276,277]. Prostaglandins and thromboxanes contain a characteristic cyclopentane ring between C_8 and C_{12} which is not present in leukotrienes and H(P)ETEs [278].

Briefly, the enzymatic pathway for membrane phospholipid-derivatives starts with a cleavage by phospholipase A_2 (PLA_2) of each phospholipid molecule into two sets of mediators: the larger part becomes PAF whereas the smaller is known as arachidonic acid [275]. Subsequently, the arachidonic acid can be processed along two pathways: the cyclooxygenase (COX) pathway, which leads to the prostaglandins and thromboxanes, and the 5-lipoxygenase (5-LO) pathway, which produces the leukotrienes [279]. The initial step in the cascade is a receptor-mediated influx of intracellular $[Ca^{2+}]_i$ (caused by e.g. zymosan) which activates cytosolic PLA_2 and induces its translocation to the nuclear envelope and endoplasmic reticulum [280]. However, there are also alternative non-$[Ca^{2+}]_i$-dependent pathways for regulating $cPLA_2$ [281]. Cyclooxygenase and 5-lipoxygenase are also localized to these sites upon activation by calcium ions [282]. Additionally, 5-lipoxygenase activating protein (FLAP) increases activity of 5-LO [283].

Although, eicosanoids are not stored as preformed mediators but are synthesized *de novo* upon stimulation, they can be produced and released within minutes [284]. This is due to constitutive expression of key enzymes: 5-lipoxygenase and cyclooxygenase (i.e. prostaglandin G/H synthase; PGHS) [285]. The latter enzyme exists in two isoforms, COX-1/PGHS-1 (constitutive) and COX-2/ PGHS-2 (inducible) [286-288]. Both enzymes carry out an identical catalytic activity and have a similar primary protein structure (75% homologous) [289] but they differ in mRNA stability and utilization of arachidonic acid pools [290]. COX-1 appears to function in both physiological ("housekeeping") and pathological systems but the other isomer (COX-2) is implicated in the formation of inflammatory mediators [291]. Thus, the production of prostaglandins in response to stimuli can be either immediate (minutes to 1 hour) or delayed (hours) when mediated by COX-1 and COX-2, respectively [292]. However, COX-2-mediated immediate prostaglandin production can be observed in cells constitutively expressing this isoform (i.e. tumors) [293,294]. Moreover, overexpression of COX-2 was recently reported in numerous healthy tissues including vascular endothelium [295,296] as well as inducible expression of COX-1 [297].

A few years ago, an existence of cyclooxygenase-3, the third isomer of COX was postulated and it was hypothesized that the putative COX-3 might be involved in a resolution of inflammation [286]. In fact, two years later Chandrasekharan et al. [298] described a new COX activity in dogs – and the discovered molecule was subsequently named cyclooxygenase 3 (COX-3); however, the described COX turned out to be something else than that predicted earlier as it was neither selectively inhibited by paracetamol nor related structurally to COX-2 and anti-inflammatory [287,288,299].

In contrast to cyclooxygenase, 5-lipoxygenase exists only in one form and is expressed exclusively in myeloid cells, e.g. monocytes, macrophages and mast cells, which differ in the type and quantity of produced leukotrienes [300].

The action of eicosanoids and PAF is mediated by specific G protein-coupled receptors with seven transmembrane domains [301,302]. All prostaglandins, PAF and cysteinyl-leukotrienes (Cys-LT; LTC_4, LTD_4, and LTE_4) participate in mediating the increase of vascular permeability but they can act in various ways. They can either act on vascular endothelium inducing contraction of smooth muscle (vasoconstriction) or increase blood flow through vessels (vasodilatation) and thereby increase the exudation of fluid [303]. The latter event may occur with or without the direct increase of vascular leakage [1].

In the course of inflammation, eicosanoids and PAF contribute not only to *rubor* and *tumor* (via vasodilatation) but also *dolor* (pain) as some of these mediators are involved in the development of hyperalgesia [284]. Moreover, PGE_2 is also a potent pyrogenic agent and thereby causes fever (*calor*) [304].

4.5. Chemokines

Chemokines and other chemoattractants (i.e. LTB_4, PAF, complement factor C5a) play a crucial role in the above process due to their ability to attract and stimulate leukocytes [305,306]. Chemokines (*chemo*attractant cyto*kines*) are small proteins that are defined by a common structural motif, i.e. possession of four cysteine residues. Chemokines are divided into two major groups, CXC (α chemokines) and CC (β chemokines) based on the presence or absence of an amino acid between the first two cysteines, respectively. More recently two other groups have been described: C that contains only two of the four cysteine residues, and CX_3C with three amino acids between cysteine residues [63,307]. CXC chemokines (e.g. IL-8=CXCL8; MIP-2α=CXCL2) show selectivity toward neutrophils while CC chemokines (e.g. MCP-1=CCL2, MIP-1β=CCL4, RANTES=CCL5) affect monocytes and also eosinophils, lymphocytes and neutrophils [54,306].

In the process of leukocyte recruitment chemokines can participate on at least three levels since they up-regulate leukocytic β_2 integrins [308] and cause selective accumulation of leukocytes [309]. Finally, chemokines can activate leukocytes once they arrive at their destination as they can trigger release of destructive enzymes and stimulate respiratory burst [310].

Recent studies indicate that chemokines are not direct-acting agents but act via mast cell-derived mediators [54]. It was demonstrated that IL-8-induced neutrophil accumulation relied on endogenous histamine [311]. The induction of leukocyte accumulation through resident mast cells was also demonstrated in action of MCP-1 and MIP-1α [162,312]. Thus, Perretti [54] suggested that chemokines operate through a mechanism in which firstly mast cell-derived histamine promotes contact (by up-regulating P-selectins) between leukocytes and endothelial cells, and subsequently the endothelium presents the direct-acting chemokine to the leukocyte.

4.6. Pro-Inflammatory Cytokines

Both the resident and the infiltrating cells produce and release cytokines upon inflammatory activation. Cytokines are a group of potent polypeptides produced by various cell types, which act in a paracrine (short-range), autocrine (on itself), or endocrine (hormone-like) fashion to modify and modulate immune and inflammatory reactions [119]. Several cytokines play key roles in mediating acute inflammatory reactions, constituting three major groups: pro-inflammatory (TNF-α, IL-1β, IL-6), chemotactic (IL-8, MCP-1, MIP), and anti-inflammatory (IL-4, IL-10, IL-13, TGF-β) cytokines [119,313,314].

Tumor necrosis factor alpha (TNF-α) and interleukin-1 (IL-1) are immediately released in response to inflammatory stimuli, as they are stored in mast cell granules. However, they are produced in greatest amounts by activated Mø, neutrophils and endothelial cells [313]. The TNF-α is the first inflammatory cytokine to be produced *de novo* and it induces subsequent synthesis of IL-1 [315,316] (Figure 4). The TNF-α (157 amino acid protein) is structurally and functionally related to lymphotoxin (i.e. TNF-β), a protein typically produced by activated lymphocytes [317]. The TNF-α exerts its effects by binding, as a trimer, to either a 55 kDa cell membrane receptor termed TNFRI or a 75 kDa cell membrane receptor termed TNFRII. Both these receptors belong to the so-called TNF receptor superfamily, including also Fas and CD40 [318]. The membrane-associated form of TNF-α can be cleaved by TNF-α-converting enzyme (TACE), a member of metalloproteinase family, to generate soluble TNF-α [319].

The Interleukin-1 family includes IL-α and IL-β that show 26% homology between their amino acid sequences and are encoded by two different genes [320]. Their size ranges from 22-31 kDa for cell-assosiated molecules, and 17.5 kDa for the secreted molecule [321]. The IL-α and IL-β act by binding to a common receptor, the type I IL-1 (IL-1RI), and a required signaling component, the IL-1R accessory protein (AcP) [320,322]). Additional regulation is provided by the type II, or decoy, IL-1 receptor (IL-1RII), which binds and sequesters IL-1β (mainly), without inducing any signaling response of its own [323]. The receptors belong to the Immunoglobulin (Ig)- superfamily that also includes adhesion molecules and MHCs [324]. Interleukin-1α and IL-1β share similar biological activities, although IL-1α remains mostly membrane associated or within cells, while IL-1β is usually secreted [320,325]; the two forms also display a distinct pattern of organ distribution [326]. Precursor IL-1α is fully functional whereas pro-IL-1β is biologically inactive [325]. Thus, specific intracellular enzyme Caspase-1, known also as IL-1β-converting enzyme (ICE), cleaves and activates pro-IL-1β into an active form [327]. The same enzyme converts pro-IL-18 into IL-18 (formerly: IFN-γ-inducing factor) that is a new member of the IL-1 family, as it resembles IL-1β in terms of both structure and function [328]. However, other enzymes, in addition to caspase-1, are able to cleave pro-IL-1β, but not pro-IL-18, and generate biologically active molecules [329]. The activity of mature IL-18 includes induction of gene expression and synthesis of TNF-α, IL-1, and several chemokines (e.g. IL-8) that places IL-18 in a strategic role in inflammation [330]. Interleukin-18 also participates in acquired immunity as, for example, it induces production of IFN-γ from activated Th_1 cells and stimulates their proliferation and cytotoxicity [331].

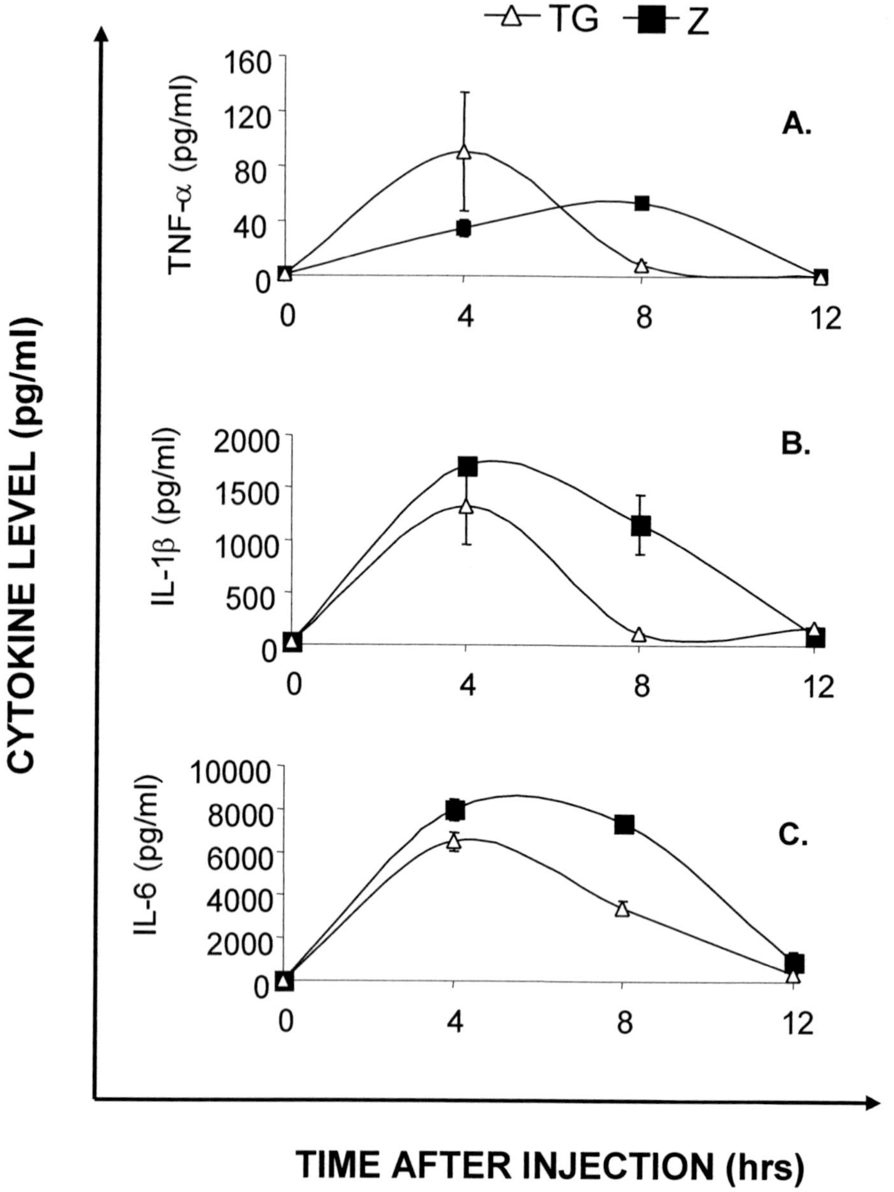

Figure 4. Kinetics of proinflammatory cytokine levels in peritoneal fluid in male Swiss mice. Animals were i.p. injected with either 3% thioglycollate – TG or zymosan – Z (2mg/ml; 0.5 ml/mouse) and sacrificed at the selected time points after treatment; time 0 – intact animals. Peritoneal cavity was lavaged with 1 ml of saline and (A) TNF-α, (B) IL-1β and (C) IL-6 content was estimated in peritoneal fluid by ELISAs. Means ± SE, n=4-8.

Functionally, TNF-α and IL-1β are closely related, although their respective structures and the specific receptors are clearly distinct [119]. They act synergistically to induce the expression of chemokines and up-regulate cell adhesion molecules and thus trigger leukocyte emigration to the inflammatory site [332]. The TNF-α and IL-1β are also potent inducers of phospholipase A_2 (PLA_2) and cyclooxygenase-2 (COX-2) enzymes responsible for production of lipid mediators [333]. Interleukin-1 can also elicit the release of histamine from mast cells and thus trigger the increase of vascular permeability [334]. TNF-α and IL-1β further exert secondary inflammatory effects by stimulating IL-6 synthesis (Figure 4), which in turn continues to mediate their actions by, for example, induction of fever and stimulation of acute phase protein synthesis in liver [335].

5. SICKNESS

As we indicated above, TNF-α, IL-1 and IL-6 released by activated leukocytes during inflammation orchestrate innate and adaptive immune responses, but they also act on the brain structures and mediate the behavioral changes named collectively "sickness behavior" [336]. Peripherally released cytokines act on the brain via a fast transmission pathway involving primery afferent nerves innervating the focus of inflammation and a slow transmission pathway involving cytokines orginating from the choroid plexus and circumventricular organs and diffusing into the brain parenchyma by volume transmission [336]. Alternatively, the cytokines can trigger a release of subsequent messengers such as cytokines from microglial cells [337] and prostaglandin E_2 (PGE_2) from brain endothelial cells [338]. In fact, in situ hybridization, immunocytochemistry and PCR studies indicated presence of mRNA for both pro-inflammatory mediator proteins and their receptors in the brain structures [339]. Pro-inflammatory mediators bound to receptors in the brain structures modulate synthesis/release of some neuropeptides and hormones [336] and as a consequence sick animals demonstrate sleepiness, reduced food and water intake, depressed locomotor and body care activity, decreased social and sexual behavior and impaired learning and memory [336]. These behavioural changes conserve the energy necessary to fight infection and reduce susceptability to predators [340].

5.1. Inflammatory Pain

During inflammation, inflammatory mediators sensitize the specialized peripheral nerve-fiber endings, and thus cause pain (Figure 5). The sensitization of nociceptors ("pain receptors") is rapidly induced and the mentioned changes can be observed within a few minutes [341,342]. The inflammatory endogenous hyperalgesic mediators that are synthesized and released in the early stages of inflammation include pro-inflammatory cytokines (TNF α, IL-1, IL-6) (Figure 4), prostaglandins (mainly PGI_2), bradikinin, histamine and nerve growth factor [1,3,29,341,343]. Simultaneously, the expression of receptors for inflammatory mediators in the primary afferents is changed, e.g. during arthritis in the rat the expression of bradikinin receptors in dorsal root ganglia and in peripheral nerve fibers is enhanced [344]. Furthermore, inflammation reduces threshold of nociceptor excitation thus the normally insensible factors such as light can also induce pain [342].

For example, early stages of murine zymosan-induced peritonitis are connected with visceral pain response (writhing) (Figure 5), consisting of a contraction of the abdominal muscles together with a stretching of hind limbs and sedation [3,29,345]. The frequency of writhes turned out to be strain-dependent [345,346] (Figure 9A), but in general the writhes are restricted to the first thirty minutes after zymosan injection.

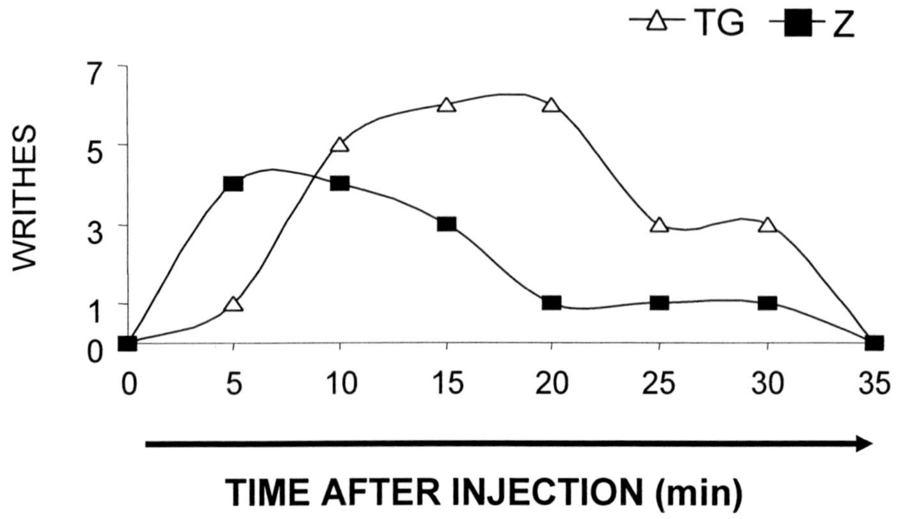

Figure 5. Nociceptive activity of male Swiss mice i.p. injected with either 3% thioglycollate – TG or zymosan – Z (2mg/ml; 0.5 ml/mouse). Characteristic body writhes (consisting of a contraction of the abdominal muscles together with a stretching of hind limbs) were counted during five-minute intervals for each mouse (all together during thirthy five minutes). Representative data from one individual.

5.2. Participation of Endogenous Opioids

The important role in the control of inflammatory pain is played by endogenous opioid peptides such as endorphins, enkephalins and dynorphins. As evidenced in series of experiments on Freund's complete adjuvant-induced paw inflammation in the rat, inflammation induces up-regulation of opioid receptors on the local peripheral endings of sensory neurons and increases levels of the opioid peptides in inflammatory leukocytes e.g. [347-350]. Opioid peptides are synthesized within various types of immune cells and are released locally in the inflamed tissue [341]. Binding of opioid peptides to their receptors on peripheral sensory neurons results in potent analgesia [347-349].

The results of our experiments on zymosan-induced peritoneal inflammation in mice suggest dual origin of the opioid peptides accumulating in the focus of inflammation, which may derive from exudatory leukocytes and from distal neurohormonal centres. During peritonitis, exudatory peritoneal leukocytes express elevated levels of mRNAs for the precursor molecules of proopiomelanocortin (POMC), proenkephalin (PENK) and prodynorphin (PDYN) (Figure 6), thus exudatory leukocytes may be a source of opioid peptides released into peritoneal fluid [351-354] (Figure 7). On the other hand, in parallel with the increase of met-enkephalin levels in the peritoneal fluid the rapid reduction of its levels was recorded in striatum and hypothalamus [352,354] (Figure 8).

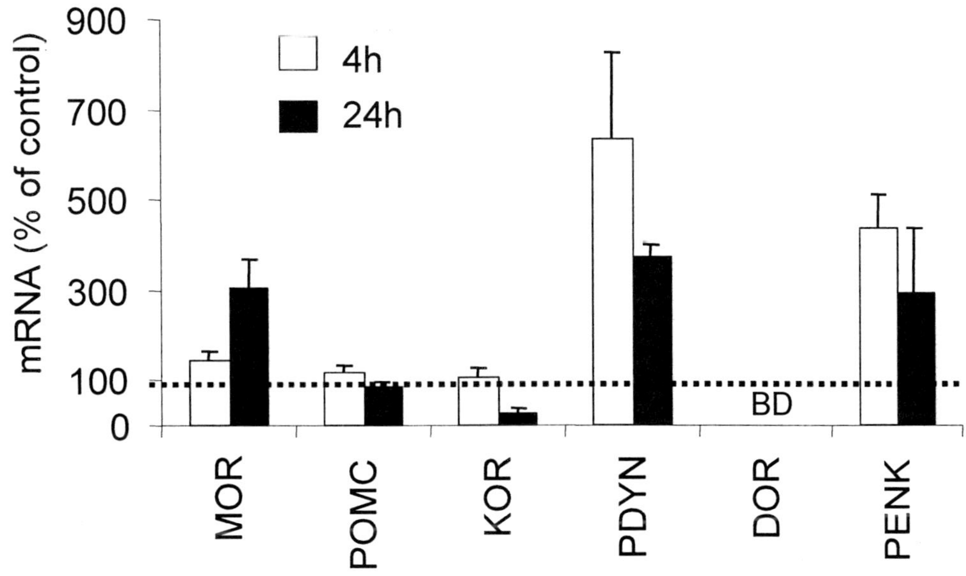

Figure 6. Alternation in expression of mRNA for opioid receptors: mu (MOR), kappa (KOR) and delta (DOR), and opioid prohormones: proopiomelanocortin (POMC), prodynorphin (PDYN) and proenkephalin (PENK) in pellets of peritoneal leukocytes retrieved from male Swiss mice. Animals were i.p. injected with zymosan – Z (2mg/ml; 0.5 ml/mouse) and sacrificed 4 or 24 hrs after irritant injection; peritoneal cavities were lavaged with 1 ml of saline, subsequently exudates were centrifuged and total mRNA was extracted according to Chomczynski method [383] from leukocytes pelet and measured by quantitative real-time detection (for method see [351]). The results were recalculated as a percentage of control (dashed line), means ± SE, n=4-8. BD – expression below detection.

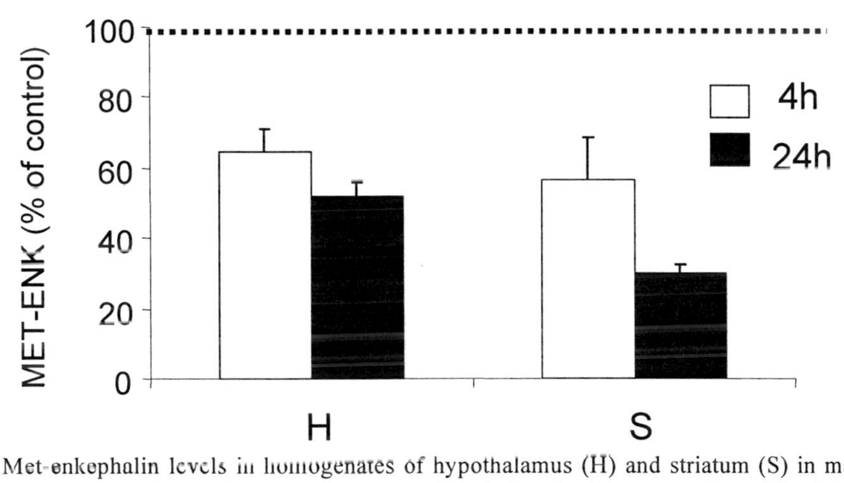

Figure 8. Met-enkephalin levels in homogenates of hypothalamus (H) and striatum (S) in male Swiss mice. Animals were i.p. injected with zymosan – Z (2mg/ml; 0.5 ml/mouse) and sacrificed 4 or 24 hrs after injection. Met-enkephalin levels were measured by competitive radioimmunoassay (RIA) (for method see [384]) and the results were recalculated as a percentage of control (dashed line). Means ± SE, n=4-8.

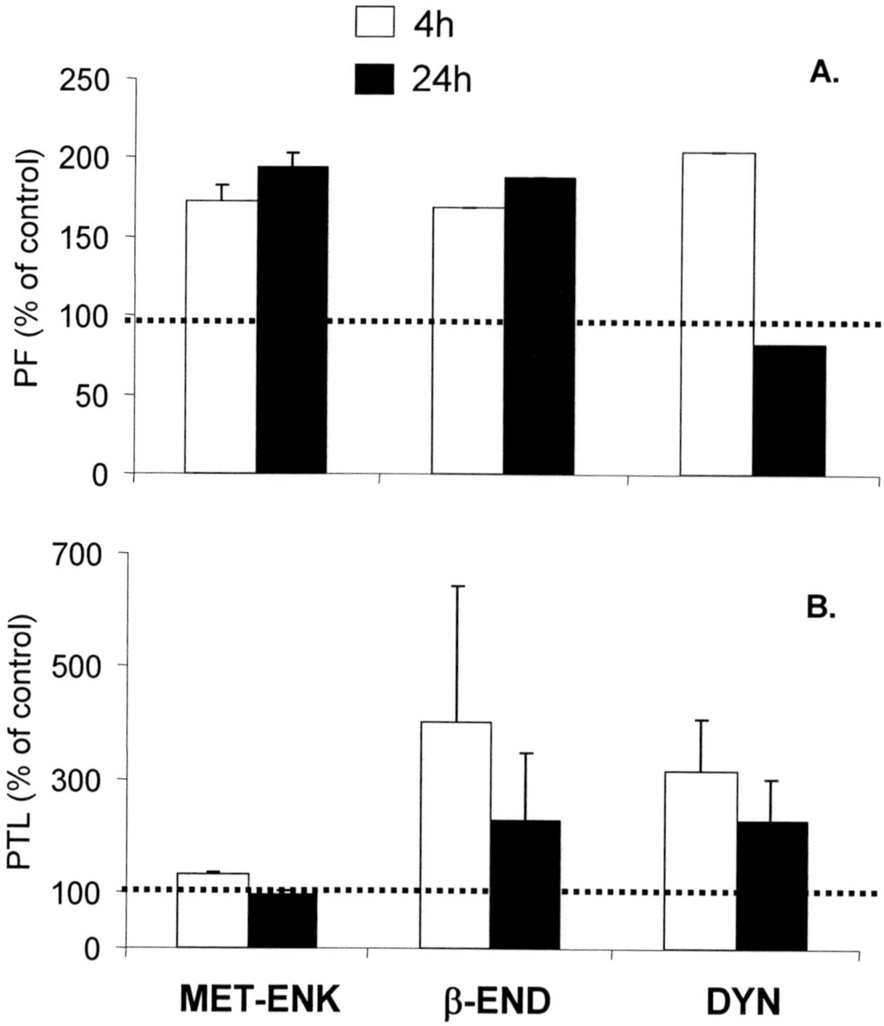

Figure 7. Alternation in the level of met-enkephalin (MET-ENK), β-endorfin (β-END) and dynorphin (DYN) in (A) peritoneal fluid (PF) and (B) in total pelet of peritoneal leukocytes (PTL) in male Swiss mice. Animals were i.p. injected with zymosan – Z (2mg/ml; 0.5 ml/mouse) and sacrificed 4 or 24 hrs after irritant injection. Opioid peptide levels were measured by competitive radioimmunoassay (RIA) (for method see [384]) and the results were recalculated as a percentage of control (dashed line). Means ± SE, n=4-8.

Furthermore, we also observed inflammation-induced changes in expression of mu and kappa opioid receptors on peritoneal leukocytes [351] (Figure 6). The presence of opiod receptors on immunocompetent cells (e.g. [355,356]) indicates an importance of opioid system in the immunoregulation [357]. Studies from several laboratories suggest that opioids can act as very potent communication signals of the immune system and as such can be included among cytokines [358].

5.3. Effects of Exogenous Opioids

In the light of proved crucial involvement of endogenous opioids and their receptors in the control of inflammatory pain it seems obvious that exogenous morphine should also affect inflammatory pain. In fact, supplementation of inflammation-inducing irritant with morphine abolishes in mice pain symptoms (writhes) (Figure 9A). Interestingly, in several strains of mice: Swiss, C57BL, Balb/c (but not in CBA), a high dose of morphine (20mg/kg) additionally suppressed leukocyte accumulation in the focus of inflammation (Figures 9B, 10C).

The similar phenomenon was also observed in the investigated teleost fish, Atlantic salmon [33], and goldfish [34] (Figure 10A), but not in several investigated anuran amphibian species [38] (e.g Figure 10B).

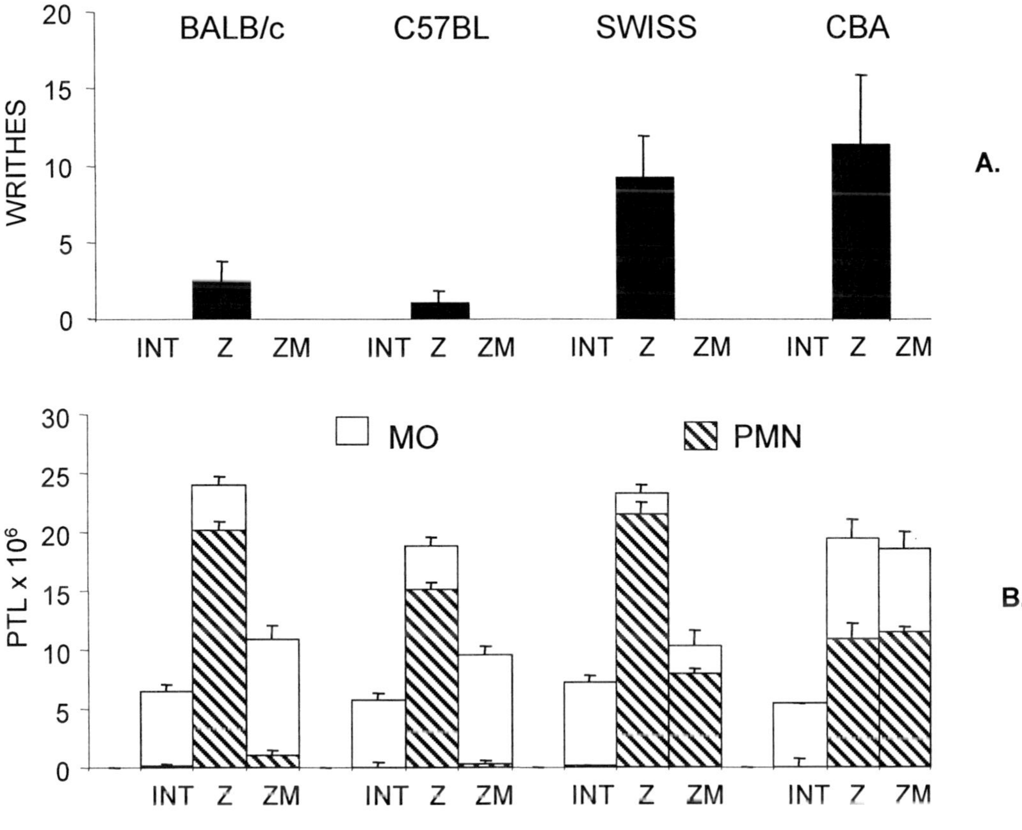

Figure 9. Effects of morphine on the number of (A) pain symptoms – body writhes and (B) peritoneal leukocytes (PTL) in several strains of mice. Animals were i.p. injected with either zymosan (2mg/ml; 0.5 ml/mouse; Z) or zymosan supplemented with morphine hydrochloride (20mg/kg b.w.; ZM). Characteristic body writhes (consisting of a contraction of the abdominal muscles together with a stretching of hind limbs) were counted during 35 minutes after injection. Mice were sacrificed at time 0 (intact – INT) or 4 hrs after Z or ZM injection. Peritoneal cavity was lavaged with 1 ml of saline and the number of mononuclear (MO) and polymorphonuclear (PMN) leukocytes was counted with a hemocytometer following staining with Turk's solutions (0.01% crystal violet in 3% acetic acid). Means ± SE, n=4-8.

We suppose that morphine-insensitivity of amphibians might be connected with the presence of high levels of unique endogenous opiods, deltorphine and dermorphine in these animals [359].

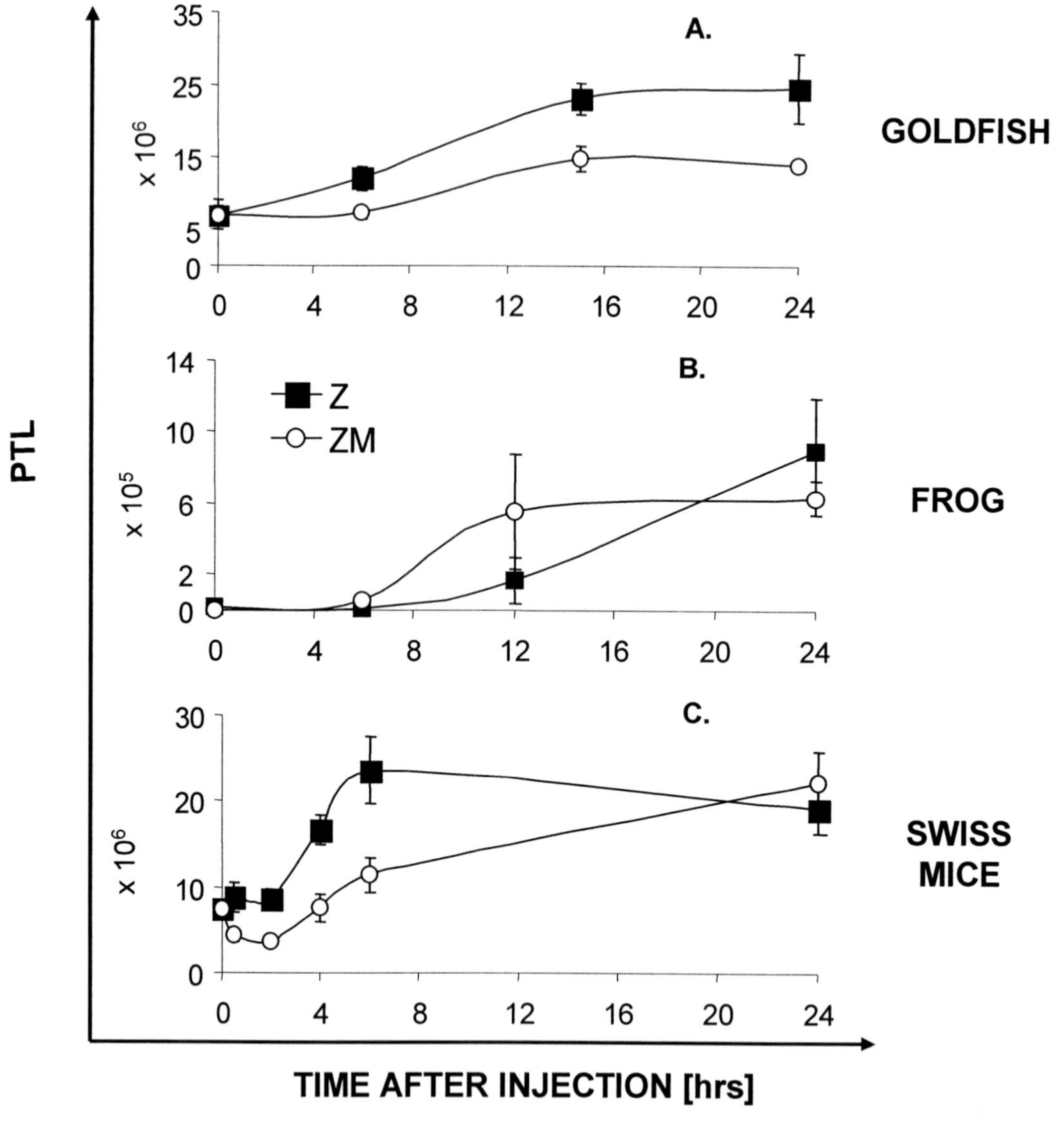

Figure 10. Effects of morphine on peritoneal inflammation in (A) goldfish (*Carassius auratus*), (B) edible frog (*Rana esculenta*) and (C) Swiss mice. Animals were i.p. injected with either zymosan (2mg/ml; 0.5 ml/mouse; Z) or zymosan supplemented with morphine hydrochloride (20mg/kg b.w.; ZM) and sacrificed at the selected time points after treatment; time 0 – intact animals. Peritoneal cavity was lavaged with 1 ml of saline and the total number of peritoneal leukocytes (PTL) was counted with a hemocytometer. Means ± SE, n=4-8. In a case of CBA mice the lack of morphine effects on inflammation can be explained by the abundance of peritoneal mast cells and sensitivity of their mast cells to morphine-induced degranulation, characteristic feature of this strain of mice [360].

The important role of mast cells in morphine-mediated inhibition of peritonitis is confirmed by the observation that this phenomenon is absent in mast cell-knockout mice (WBB6F1-W/W^{v}) [361] as well as in animals pre-injected with a well-known mast cell degranulator, compound 48/80 [360,361]. Interestingly, the resident macrophages are not involved in morphine-induced inhibition of peritonitis [362].

Despite reduced numbers of peritoneal leukocytes in mice injected with zymosan supplemented with morphine, kinetics of changes of pro-inflammatory cytokines (IL-1β, TNF-α, IL-6, IL-10, mKC, MCP-1) in peritoneal fluid was similar to that in mice injected with irritant only [363]. We can speculate that morphine supplementation of an irritant affects leukocyte chemotactic response as it induces the reduction of some chemotactic factors both in the peritoneal fluid and blood plasma [33,362,363] and/or heterologous desensitization of some leukocyte receptors for chemoattractants [364-367]. However, we cannot exclude a possibility that morphine also induces apoptosis of resident and exudatory leukocytes since the pro-apoptotic effects of morphine were observed under *in vitro* condition e.g. in murine macrophage cell line J774 [368,369].

6. Comparative Studies on Peritonitis

Experimental peritonitis is convenient for comparative studies on inflammatory processes in all vertebrates, both endothermic mammals and ectothermic fish and amphibians. It turned out that a course of inflammation is species- and strain-specific and varies according to the age and sex of experimental animals as well as according to the kind and dose of stimulus used [38,346,370-372].

6.1. Peritonitis in Ectothermic Animals

The ectothermic animals, such as fish and amphibians, offer possibility to study effects of ambient temperature on the course of inflammation. It turned out that the low temperature affects intraperitoneal accumulation of leukocytes in a species-specific manner. In the goldfish (*Carassius auratus*) and the edible frog (*Rana esculenta*), thioglycollate-induced intraperitoneal accumulation of leukocytes was massive and relatively short-lasting at the room temperature. However, intraperitoneal influx of leukocytes at 10°C was completely inhibited in the goldfish, while in the edible frog was significantly delayed and prolonged (Figure 11). It turned out, however, that the duration of inflammation was also significantly prolonged in the grass frog, *Rana temporaria*, kept at the room temperature during the winter in comparison with the vigorous inflammatory process in animals investigated during the summer (Figure 12 B), indicating the existence of the endogenous annual rhythm of immunity [373]. On the other hand, at the same season the adult frogs react much more vigorously then the juveniles of the same species (Figure 12 A).

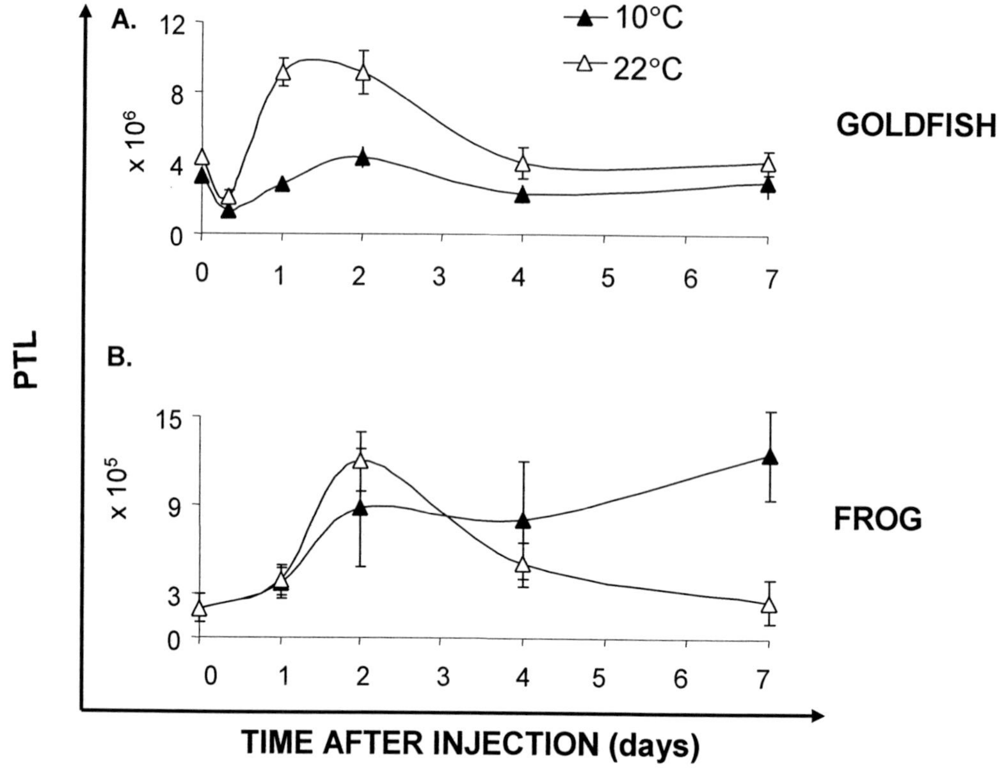

Figure 11. Effects of ambient temperature (10°C or 22°C) on peritoneal inflammation in juvenile individuals of (A) goldfish (*Carassius auratus*) and (B) edible frog (*Rana esculenta*). Animals were i.p. injected with 3% thioglycollate and sacrificed at the selected time points after treatment; time 0 – intact animals. Peritoneal cavity was lavaged with saline and the total number of peritoneal leukocytes (PTL) and was counted with a hemocytometer. Means ± SE, n=3-12.

6.2. Effects of Stress on Peritonitis

In the field-collected amphibians or in the fish delivered from the fish farm the course of inflammation may be also affected by uncontrolled previous life events of investigated animals. It turned out, however, that the kinetics of inflammation may be unintentionally modified by some factors connected with an experimental procedure. For example, sterile pre-injection of physiological saline or even sterile puncture or handling of experimental animals may modify the early stages of the subsequently evoked peritoneal inflammation [374,375]. Also it turned out that mice delivered by various suppliers differ in the reaction to the same pro-inflammatory stimulus [370]. Besides minor genetic differences between animals bred by various suppliers, this discrepancy may be caused by a social stress connected with transportation and changes in housing conditions. This could explain the variations between different sets of experiments performed by the same investigators on laboratory strains of mice carefully matched according to age and gender under the same laboratory conditions. As a rule numerous mice share the same large cages during transportation. After arrival the even numbers of cage-mates are distributed to the final cages and allowed to adapt for at least one week to the strictly controlled light, humidity, and housing conditions in the new animal facilities [5,33,353,376].

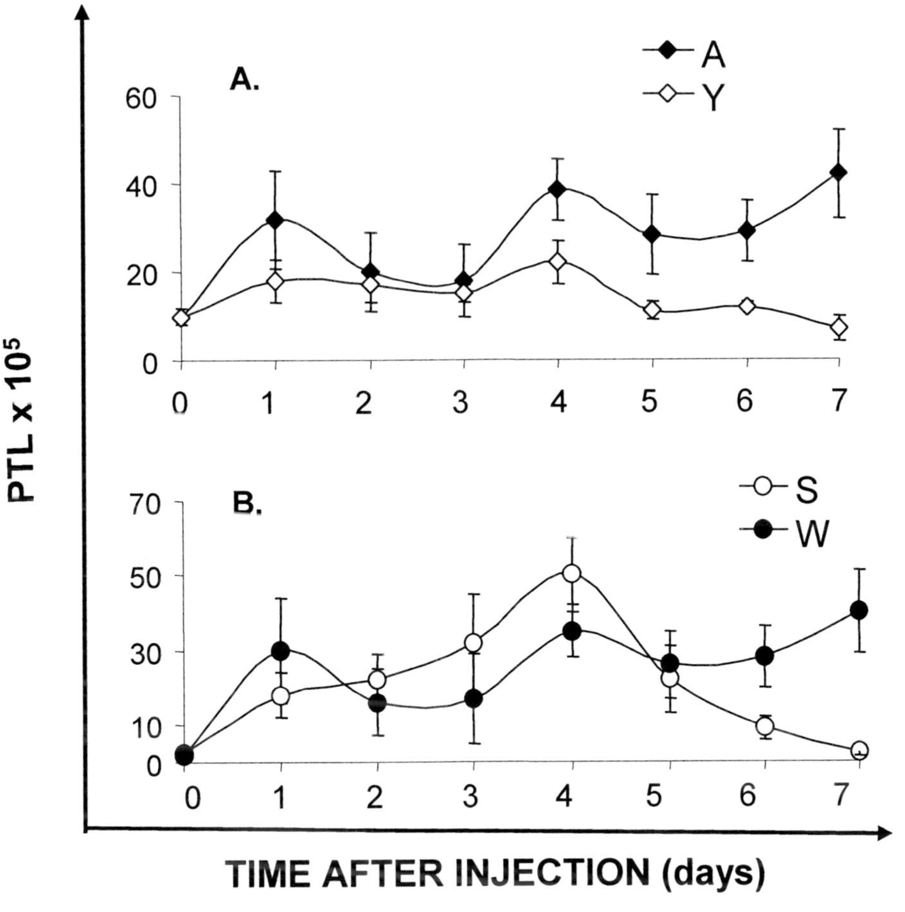

Figure 12. Effects of age (A) and season (B) on peritoneal inflammation in grass frog (*Rana temporaria*). Animals were i.p. injected with sephadex G-50 (100ml/kg b.w.) and sacrificed at the selected time points after treatment; time 0 – intact animals. Peritoneal cavity was lavaged with saline and the total number of peritoneal leukocytes (PTL) was counted with a hemocytometer. The minimum age of animals was estimated by counting the annual rings of hematoxyline-stained cross-sections throug femurs, Y – young frogs, A – adult frogs, W - winter, S - summer. Means ± SE, n=3-10.

We have shown that the social stress of isolation or grouping of mice may affect various inflammation-related factors, e.g. pain symptoms and leukocyte accumulation (Figure 13), in a strain-dependent manner in C57C3H, Swiss, and Balb/c males. In contrast, males of C57/BL were resistant to a social stress [371], which corresponds with their resistance to stress induced by odor of foot-shocked conspecific animals [377].

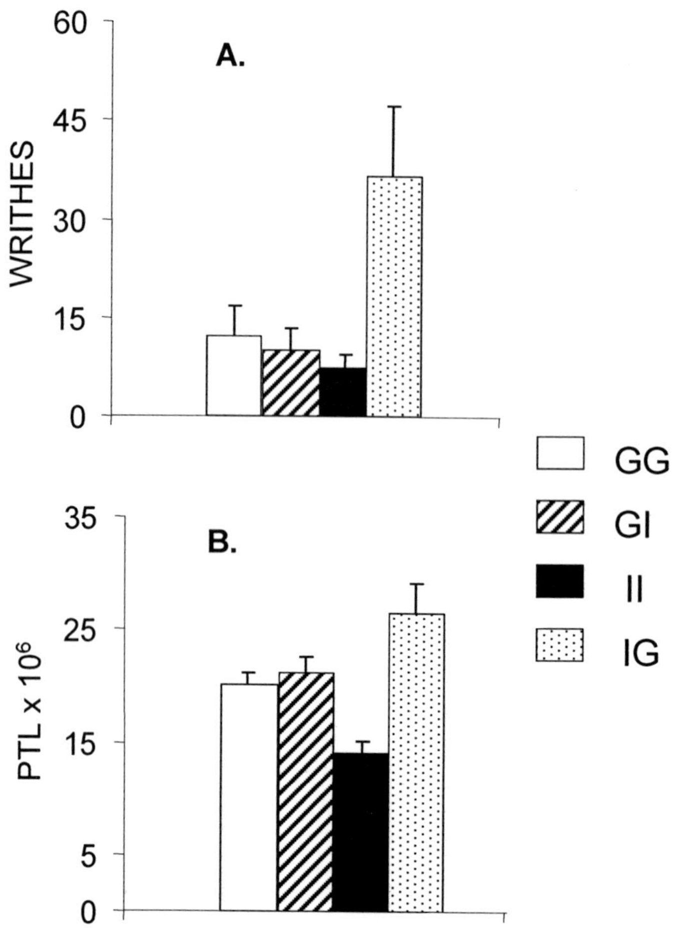

Figure 13. Effect of social stress connected with a change of housing condition (isolation or grouping) of the male Swiss mice on the number of (A) pain symptoms - writhes and (B) peritoneal cell number (PTL) during peritoneal inflammation in male Swiss mice. Animals were housed 4 per cage (GG), 1 per cage (II) or shifted from group to isolation (GI) or from isolation to group (IG). After zymosan injection characteristic body writhes (consisting of a contraction of the abdominal muscles together with a stretching of hind limbs) were counted during 35 minutes after injection. Animals were sacrificed 4 hrs after irritant injection and peritoneal cavities were lavaged with 1 ml of saline. PTLs were counted with a hemocytometer. Means ± SE, n=4-8.

7. Conclusion: Inflammation as a Part of Homeostatic System of the Body

Homeostasis of an organism dependends on multi-directional communication between the cells of the nervous, endocrine, and immune systems that share receptors and mediators [378]. They monitor the environment to give adaptive responses to psychical or physical disturbances, including pathogenic infections. In the latter case the inflammatory response develops that may be considered as a stress response with a pathogen being a stressor [379]. This point of view is straightened by results showing elevated levels of corticosteroids during inflammatory response in both endothermic and ectothermic animals (Figure 14). Such an antigen-induced stress response may be modified by other stressing events (see [379]). As mentioned above, cytokines produced during inflammation act not only locally but affect the central nervous system and induce changes called "sickness behaviour" such as depression of animal mobility, decreased exploration of physical and social environment, reduced food and water intake, and impaired learning and memory [380]. The recent findings of mechanisms operating during inflammation must be interpreted in the context of the environment in which animals and human live [381,382].

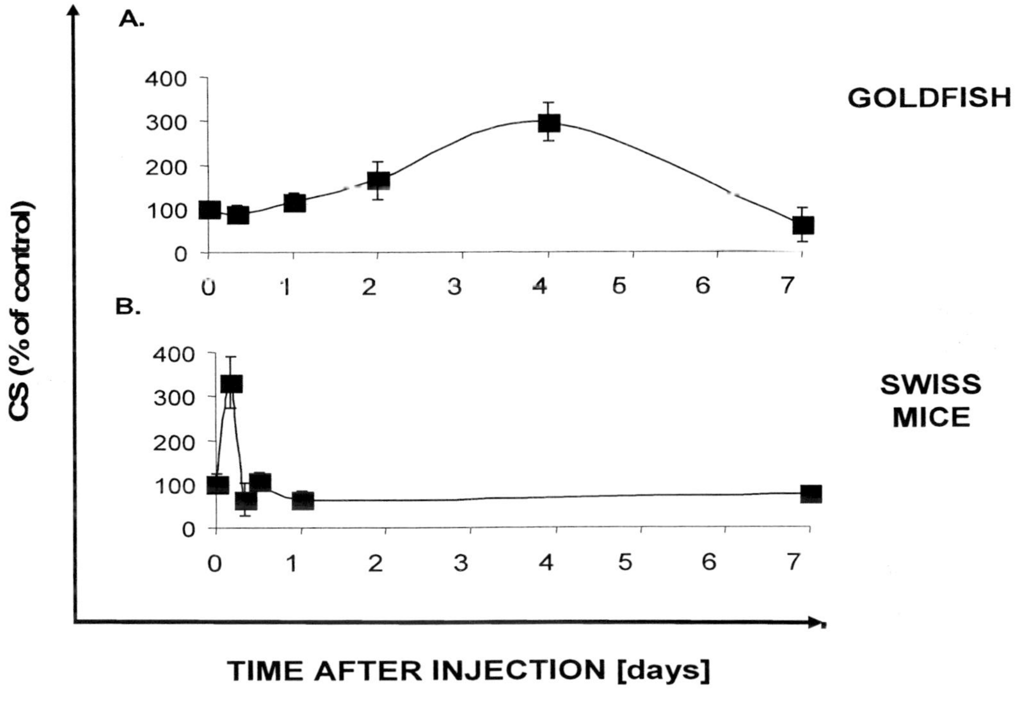

Figure 14. Kinetics of blood corticosteroids levels (CS) during zymosan-induced peritonitis; (A) cortisol levels in goldfish (*Carassius auratus*) and (B) corticosterone levels in Swiss mice. Animals were i.p. injected with zymosan – Z (2mg/ml; 0.5 ml/mouse) and sacrificed at the selected time points after irritant injection; time 0 – intact animals. Corticosteroid levels were measured in blood plasma by RIA, and the results were recalculated as a percentage of control. Means ± SE, n=4-8.

REFERENCES

[1] Majno, G., Joris, I. (1996) *Cells, tissues, and disease: principles of general pathology.* Blackwell, Oxford.

[2] Kolaczkowska, E. (2001) Experimental acute peritonitis and its modulation by morphine: involvement of mast cells and macrophages. *Ph.D. thesis*, University of Tromso, Norway.

[3] Doherty, N.S., Poubelle, P., Borgeat, P., Beaver, T.H., Westrich, G.L., Schrader, N.L. (1985) Intraperitoneal injection of zymosan in mice induces pain, inflammation and the synthesis of peptidoleukotrienes and prostaglandin E2. *Prostaglandins 30*, 769-89.

[4] Doherty, N.S., Griffiths, R.J., Hakkinen, J.P., Scampoli, D.N., Milici, A.J. (1995) Post-capillary venules in the "milky spots" of the greater omentum are the major site of plasma protein and leukocyte extravasation in rodent models of peritonitis. *Inflamm Res 44*, 169-77.

[5] Kolaczkowska, E., Seljelid, R., Plytycz, B. (2001) Role of mast cells in zymosan-induced peritoneal inflammation in Balb/c and mast cell-deficient WBB6F1 mice. *J Leukoc Biol 69*, 33-42.

[6] Kolaczkowska, E., Shahzidi, S., Seljelid, R., van Rooijen, N., Plytycz, B. (2002) Early vascular permeability in murine experimental peritonitis is comediated by resident peritoneal macrophages and mast cells: crucial involvement of macrophage-derived cysteinyl-leukotrienes. *Inflammation 26*, 61-71.

[7] Kolaczkowska, E. (2002) Shedding light on vascular permeability during peritonitis: role of mast cell histamine versus macrophage cysteinyl leukotrienes. *Inflamm Res 51*, 519-21.

[8] Lurie, M.B. (1964) *Resistance to tuberculosis: experimental studies in native and acquired defensive mechanisms*. Harvard University Press, Cambridge.

[9] Adams, D.O. (1983) The biology of granuloma. In *Pathology of granuloma* (H. I. Ioachim, ed) Raven Press, New York 1-20.

[10] Lo, D., Feng, L., Li, L., Carson, M.J., Crowley, M., Pauza, M., Nguyen, A., Reilly, C.R. (1999) Integrating innate and adaptive immunity in the whole animal. *Immunol Rev 169*, 225-39.

[11] Majno, G. (1982) Inflammation and infection: historic highlights. In *Current topics in inflammation and infection* (G. Majno, R. S. Cotran and N. Kaufman, eds.), Williams and Wilkins, Baltimore 1-17.

[12] Cohnheim, J. (1867) Ueber Entzundung und Eiterung. *Virchows Arch. Pathol. Anat. Physiol. Klin. Med. 40*, 1-79.

[13] Metchnikoff, E. (1884) Ueber eine Sprosspilzkrankheit der Daphnien. Beitrag zur Lehre uber den Kampf der Phagocyten gegen Krankheitserreger. *Virchows Arch. Pathol. Anat. Physiol. Klin. Med. 96*, 177-195.

[14] Metchnikoff, E. (1893) *Lecons sur la pathologie comparee de l'inflammation. Masson, Paris. Reissued in English as Lectures on comparative pathology of inflammation (translated from French by F.A. Starling and E.H. Starling, MD).* Reproduced by Dover Publications, Inc., New York, 1986.

[15] Sedgwick, A.D., Lees, P. (1986) A comparison of air pouch, sponge and pleurisy models of acute carrageenan inflammation in the rat. *Agents Actions 18*, 439-46.

[16] Dawson, J., Sedgwick, A.D., Edwards, J.C., Lees, P. (1991) A comparative study of the cellular, exudative and histological responses to carrageenan, dextran and zymosan in the mouse. *Int J Tissue React 13*, 171-85.

[17] Martin, S.W., Stevens, A.J., Brennan, B.S., Davies, D., Rowland, M., Houston, J.B. (1994) The six-day-old rat air pouch model of inflammation: characterization of the inflammatory response to carrageenan. *J Pharmacol Toxicol Methods 32*, 139-47.

[18] Paya, M., Garcia Pastor, P., Coloma, J., Alcaraz, M.J. (1997) Nitric oxide synthase and cyclo-oxygenase pathways in the inflammatory response induced by zymosan in the rat air pouch. *Br J Pharmacol 120*, 1445-52.

[19] Calhoun, W., Chang, J., Carlson, R.P. (1987) Effect of selected antiinflammatory agents and other drugs on zymosan, arachidonic acid, PAF and carrageenan induced paw edema in the mouse. *Agents Actions 21*, 306-9.

[20] Henriques, M.G., Silva, P.M., Martins, M.A., Flores, C.A., Cunha, F.Q., Assreuy-Filho, J., Cordeiro, R.S. (1987) Mouse paw edema. A new model for inflammation? *Braz J Med Biol Res 20*, 243-9.

[21] Cuzzocrea, S., Costantino, G., Mazzon, E., Zingarelli, B., De Sarro, A., Caputi, A.P. (1999) Protective effects of Mn(III)tetrakis (4-benzoic acid) porphyrin (MnTBAP), a superoxide dismutase mimetic, in paw oedema induced by carrageenan in the rat. *Biochem Pharmacol 58*, 171-6.

[22] Villa, P., Sartor, G., Angelini, M., Sironi, M., Conni, M., Gnocchi, P., Isetta, A.M., Grau, G., Buurman, W., van Tits, L.J., et al. (1995) Pattern of cytokines and pharmacomodulation in sepsis induced by cecal ligation and puncture compared with that induced by endotoxin. *Clin Diagn Lab Immunol 2*, 549-53.

[23] Matsukawa, A., Hogaboam, C.M., Lukacs, N.W., Lincoln, P.M., Evanoff, H.L., Strieter, R.M., Kunkel, S.L. (2000) Expression and contribution of endogenous IL-13 in an experimental model of sepsis. *J Immunol 164*, 2738-44.

[24] Futaki, N., Takahashi, S., Kitagawa, T., Yamakawa, Y., Tanaka, M., Higuchi, S. (1997) Selective inhibition of cyclooxygenase-2 by NS-398 in endotoxin shock rats in vivo. *Inflamm Res 46*, 496-502.

[25] Remick, D.G., Newcomb, D.E., Bolgos, G.L., Call, D.R. (2000) Comparison of the mortality and inflammatory response of two models of sepsis: lipopolysaccharide vs. cecal ligation and puncture. *Shock 13*, 110-6.

[26] Qureshi, R., Jakschik, B.A. (1988) The role of mast cells in thioglycollate-induced inflammation. *J Immunol 141*, 2090-6.

[27] Damas, J., Bourdon, V., Remacle-Volon, G., Adam, A. (1990) Kinins and peritoneal exudates induced by carrageenin and zymosan in rats. *Br J Pharmacol 101*, 418-22.

[28] Zhang, Y., Ramos, B.F., Jakschik, B.A. (1992) Neutrophil recruitment by tumor necrosis factor from mast cells in immune complex peritonitis. *Science 258*, 1957-9.

[29] Doherty, N.S., Beaver, T.H., Chan, K.Y., Dinerstein, R.J., Diekema, K.A. (1990) The antinociceptive activity of paracetamol in zymosan-induced peritonitis in mice: the role of prostacyclin and reactive oxygen species. *Br J Pharmacol 101*, 869-74.

[30] Cuzzocrea, S., Imperatore, F., Costantino, G., Luongo, C., Mazzon, E., Scafuro, M.A., Mangoni, G., Caputi, A.P., Rossi, F., Filippelli, A. (2000) Role of hyperbaric oxygen exposure in reduction of lipid peroxidation and in multiple organ failure induced by zymosan administration in the rat. *Shock 13*, 197-203.

[31] Van Der Vaart, J.M., te Biesebeke, R., Chapman, J.W., Klis, F.M., Verrips, C.T. (1996) The beta-1, 6-glucan containing side-chain of cell wall proteins of Saccharomyces

cerevisiae is bound to the glycan core of the GPI moiety. *FEMS Microbiol Lett 145*, 401-7.

[32] Ajuebor, M.N., Das, A.M., Virag, L., Flower, R.J., Szabo, C., Perretti, M. (1999) Role of resident peritoneal macrophages and mast cells in chemokine production and neutrophil migration in acute inflammation: evidence for an inhibitory loop involving endogenous IL-10. *J Immunol 162*, 1685-91.

[33] Chadzinska, M., Kolaczkowska, E., Seljelid, R., Plytycz, B. (1999) Morphine modulation of peritoneal inflammation in Atlantic salmon and CB6 mice. *J Leukoc Biol 65*, 590-6.

[34] Chadzinska, M., Scislowska-Czarnecka, A., Plytycz, B. (2000) Inhibitory effects of morphine on some inflammation-related parameters in the goldfish *Carassius auratus* L. *Fish Shellfish Immunol 10*, 531-42.

[35] Frode-Saleh, T.S., Calixto, J.B. (2000) Synergistic antiinflammatory effect of NF-kappaB inhibitors and steroidal or non steroidal antiinflammatory drugs in the pleural inflammation induced by carrageenan in mice. *Inflamm Res 49*, 330-7.

[36] Lawand, N.B., McNearney, T., Westlund, K.N. (2000) Amino acid release into the knee joint: key role in nociception and inflammation. *Pain 86*, 69-74.

[37] Matsubara, S., Nakata, A., Kikuchi, M., Kikkawa, H., Ikezawa, K., Naito, K. (1997) Strain-related differences in Sephadex bead-induced airway hyperresponsiveness and inflammation in rats. *Inflamm Res 46*, 299-305.

[38] Kolaczkowska, E., Menaszek, E., Seljelid, R., Plytycz, B. (2000) Experimental peritonitis in anuran amphibians is not suppressed by morphine treatment. *Pol J Pharmacol 52*, 323-6.

[39] Adamson, I.Y., Prieditis, H., Vincent, R. (1999) Pulmonary toxicity of an atmospheric particulate sample is due to the soluble fraction. *Toxicol Appl Pharmacol 157*, 43-50.

[40] Hiltermann, T.J., de Bruijne, C.R., Stolk, J., Zwinderman, A.H., Spieksma, F.T., Roemer, W., Steerenberg, P.A., Fischer, P.H., van Bree, L., Hiemstra, P.S. (1997) Effects of photochemical air pollution and allergen exposure on upper respiratory tract inflammation in asthmatics. *Am J Respir Crit Care Med 156*, 1765-72.

[41] Stewart, J.M. (1993) The kinin system in inflammation. *Agents Actions Suppl 42*, 145-57.

[42] O'Connor, T.M., O'Connell, J., O'Brien, D.I., Goode, T., Bredin, C.P., Shanahan, F. (2004) The role of substance P in inflammatory disease. *J Cell Physiol 201*, 167-80.

[43] Stevens, T., Garcia, J.G., Shasby, D.M., Bhattacharya, J., Malik, A.B. (2000) Mechanisms regulating endothelial cell barrier function. *Am J Physiol Lung Cell Mol Physiol 279*, L419-22.

[44] McDonald, D.M., Thurston, G., Baluk, P. (1999) Endothelial gaps as sites for plasma leakage in inflammation. *Microcirculation 6*, 7-22.

[45] Moore, T.M., Chetham, P.M., Kelly, J.J., Stevens, T. (1998) Signal transduction and regulation of lung endothelial cell permeability. Interaction between calcium and cAMP. *Am J Physiol 275*, L203-22.

[46] Stevens, T., Nakahashi, Y., Cornfield, D.N., McMurtry, I.F., Cooper, D.M., Rodman, D.M. (1995) Ca(2+)-inhibitable adenylyl cyclase modulates pulmonary artery

endothelial cell cAMP content and barrier function. *Proc Natl Acad Sci U S A 92*, 2696-700.

[47] Stevens, T., Creighton, J., Thompson, W.J. (1999) Control of cAMP in lung endothelial cell phenotypes. Implications for control of barrier function. *Am J Physiol 277*, L119-26.

[48] Tiruppathi, C., Song, W., Bergenfeldt, M., Sass, P., Malik, A.B. (1997) Gp60 activation mediates albumin transcytosis in endothelial cells by tyrosine kinase-dependent pathway. *J Biol Chem 272*, 25968-75.

[49] Majno, G., Palade, G.E. (1961) Studies on inflammation. 1. The effect of histamine and serotonin on vascular permeability: an electron microscopic study. *J Biophys Biochem Cytol 11*, 571-605.

[50] Majno, G., Palade, G.E., Schoefl, G.I. (1961) Studies on inflammation. II. The site of action of histamine and serotonin along the vascular tree: a topographic study. *J Biophys Biochem Cytol 11*, 607-26.

[51] Michel, C.C., Curry, F.E. (1999) Microvascular permeability. *Physiol Rev 79*, 703-61.

[52] Huxley, V.H., Rumbaut, R.E. (2000) The microvasculature as a dynamic regulator of volume and solute exchange. *Clin Exp Pharmacol Physiol 27*, 847-54.

[53] Szekanecz, Z., Koch, A.E. (2004) Vascular endothelium and immune responses: implications for inflammation and angiogenesis. *Rheum Dis Clin North Am 30*, 97-114.

[54] Perretti, M. (1998) Lipocortin 1 and chemokine modulation of granulocyte and monocyte accumulation in experimental inflammation. *Gen Pharmacol 31*, 545-52.

[55] Van Haastert, P.J., Devreotes, P.N. (2004) Chemotaxis: signalling the way forward. *Nat Rev Mol Cell Biol 5*, 626-34.

[56] Leirisalo-Repo, M. (1994) The present knowledge of the inflammatory process and the inflammatory mediators. *Pharmacol Toxicol 75 Suppl 2*, 1-3.

[57] Seely, A.J., Pascual, J.L., Christou, N.V. (2003) Science review: Cell membrane expression (connectivity) regulates neutrophil delivery, function and clearance. *Crit Care 7*, 291-307.

[58] Randolph, G.J., Furie, M.B. (1995) A soluble gradient of endogenous monocyte chemoattractant protein-1 promotes the transendothelial migration of monocytes in vitro. *J Immunol 155*, 3610-8.

[59] Carlos, T.M., Harlan, J.M. (1994) Leukocyte-endothelial adhesion molecules. *Blood 84*, 2068-101.

[60] Johnston, B., Butcher, E.C. (2002) Chemokines in rapid leukocyte adhesion triggering and migration. *Semin Immunol 14*, 83-92.

[61] Kishimoto, T.K., Rothlein, R. (1994) Integrins, ICAMs, and selectins: role and regulation of adhesion molecules in neutrophil recruitment to inflammatory sites. *Adv Pharmacol 25*, 117-69.

[62] Weber, C. (2003) Novel mechanistic concepts for the control of leukocyte transmigration: specialization of integrins, chemokines, and junctional molecules. *J Mol Med 81*, 4-19.

[63] Furie, M.B., Randolph, G.J. (1995) Chemokines and tissue injury. *Am J Pathol 146*, 1287-301.

[64] Dangerfield, J.P., Wang, S., Nourshargh, S. (2005) Blockade of α6 integrin inhibits IL-1β but not TNF-α-induced neutrophil transmigration in vivo. *J Leukoc Biol* 77, 159-65.

[65] Muller, W.A., Weigl, S.A., Deng, X., Phillips, D.M. (1993) PECAM-1 is required for transendothelial migration of leukocytes. *J Exp Med 178*, 449-60.

[66] Burns, A.R., Walker, D.C., Brown, E.S., Thurmon, L.T., Bowden, R.A., Keese, C.R., Simon, S.I., Entman, M.L., Smith, C.W. (1997) Neutrophil transendothelial migration is independent of tight junctions and occurs preferentially at tricellular corners. *J Immunol 159*, 2893-903.

[67] Girard, J.P., Springer, T.A. (1995) High endothelial venules (HEVs): specialized endothelium for lymphocyte migration. *Immunol Today 16*, 449-57.

[68] Tanaka, T., Ebisuno, Y., Kanemitsu, N., Umemoto, E., Yang, B.G., Jang, M.H., Miyasaka, M. (2004) Molecular determinants controlling homeostatic recirculation and tissue-specific trafficking of lymphocytes. *Int Arch Allergy Immunol 134*, 120-34.

[69] Johnston, B., Chee, A., Issekutz, T.B., Ugarova, T., Fox-Robichaud, A., Hickey, M.J., Kubes, P. (2000) Alpha 4 integrin-dependent leukocyte recruitment does not require VCAM-1 in a chronic model of inflammation. *J Immunol 164*, 3337-44.

[70] Johnston, B., Issekutz, T.B., Kubes, P. (1996) The alpha 4-integrin supports leukocyte rolling and adhesion in chronically inflamed postcapillary venules in vivo. *J Exp Med 183*, 1995-2006.

[71] Campbell, E.J., Senior, R.M., Welgus, H.G. (1987) Extracellular matrix injury during lung inflammation. *Chest 92*, 161-7.

[72] Van den Steen, P.E., Dubois, B., Nelissen, I., Rudd, P.M., Dwek, R.A., Opdenakker, G. (2002) Biochemistry and molecular biology of gelatinase B or matrix metalloproteinase-9 (MMP-9). *Crit Rev Biochem Mol Biol 37*, 375-536.

[73] Opdenakker, G., Van den Steen, P.E., Van Damme, J. (2001) Gelatinase B: a tuner and amplifier of immune functions. *Trends Immunol 22*, 571-9.

[74] Opdenakker, G., Van den Steen, P.E., Dubois, B., Nelissen, I., Van Coillie, E., Masure, S., Proost, P., Van Damme, J. (2001) Gelatinase B functions as regulator and effector in leukocyte biology. *J Leukoc Biol 69*, 851-9.

[75] Van Wart, H.E., Birkedal-Hansen, H. (1990) The cysteine switch: a principle of regulation of metalloproteinase activity with potential applicability to the entire matrix metalloproteinase gene family. *Proc Natl Acad Sci U S A 87*, 5578-82.

[76] Murphy, G., Docherty, A.J. (1992) The matrix metalloproteinases and their inhibitors. *Am J Respir Cell Mol Biol 7*, 120-5.

[77] Opdenakker, G., Van Damme, J. (1994) Cytokine-regulated proteases in autoimmune diseases. *Immunol Today 15*, 103-7.

[78] Werb, Z. (1997) ECM and cell surface proteolysis: regulating cellular ecology. *Cell 91*, 439-42.

[79] Cuzner, M.L., Opdenakker, G. (1999) Plasminogen activators and matrix metalloproteases, mediators of extracellular proteolysis in inflammatory demyelination of the central nervous system. *J Neuroimmunol 94*, 1-14.

[80] Mazzieri, R., Masiero, L., Zanetta, L., Monea, S., Onisto, M., Garbisa, S., Mignatti, P. (1997) Control of type IV collagenase activity by components of the urokinase-plasmin system: a regulatory mechanism with cell-bound reactants. *Embo J 16*, 2319-32.

[81] Kolaczkowska, E., Scislowska-Czarnecka, A., Chadzinska, M., Plytycz, B., van Rooijen, N., Opdenakker, G., Arnold, B. (2006) Enhanced early vascular permeability in gelatinase B (MMP-9)-deficient mice: putative contribution of COX-1-derived PGE2 of macrophage origin. *J Leukoc Biol 80*, 25-32.

[82] Kolaczkowska, E., Chadzinska, M., Scislowska-Czarnecka, A., Plytycz, B., Opdenakker, G., Arnold, B. (2006) Gelatinase B/matrix metalloproteinase-9 contributes to cellular infiltration in a murine model of zymosan peritonitis. *Immunobiology 211*, 137-48.

[83] Shapiro, S.D., Griffin, G.L., Gilbert, D.J., Jenkins, N.A., Copeland, N.G., Welgus, H.G., Senior, R.M., Ley, T.J. (1992) Molecular cloning, chromosomal localization, and bacterial expression of a murine macrophage metalloelastase. *J Biol Chem 267*, 4664-71.

[84] Young, R.E., Thompson, R.D., Larbi, K.Y., La, M., Roberts, C.E., Shapiro, S.D., Perretti, M., Nourshargh, S. (2004) Neutrophil elastase (NE)-deficient mice demonstrate a nonredundant role for NE in neutrophil migration, generation of proinflammatory mediators, and phagocytosis in response to zymosan particles in vivo. *J Immunol 172*, 4493-502.

[85] Shipley, J.M., Wesselschmidt, R.L., Kobayashi, D.K., Ley, T.J., Shapiro, S.D. (1996) Metalloelastase is required for macrophage-mediated proteolysis and matrix invasion in mice. *Proc Natl Acad Sci U S A 93*, 3942-6.

[86] Brew, K., Dinakarpandian, D., Nagase, H. (2000) Tissue inhibitors of metalloproteinases: evolution, structure and function. *Biochim Biophys Acta 1477*, 267-83.

[87] Cawston, T.E., Curry, V.A., Clark, I.M., Hazleman, B.L. (1990) Identification of a new metalloproteinase inhibitor that forms tight-binding complexes with collagenase. *Biochem J 269*, 183-7.

[88] Curry, T.E., Jr., Mann, J.S., Estes, R.S., Jones, P.B. (1990) Alpha 2-macroglobulin and tissue inhibitor of metalloproteinases: collagenase inhibitors in human preovulatory ovaries. *Endocrinology 127*, 63-8.

[89] Sternlicht, M.D., Werb, Z. (2001) How matrix metalloproteinases regulate cell behavior. *Annu Rev Cell Dev Biol 17*, 463-516.

[90] Shapiro, S.D., Senior, R.M. (1999) Matrix metalloproteinases. Matrix degradation and more. *Am J Respir Cell Mol Biol 20*, 1100-2.

[91] Tanaka, H., Miyazaki, N., Oashi, K., Tanaka, S., Ohmichi, M., Abe, S. (2000) Sputum matrix metalloproteinase-9: tissue inhibitor of metalloproteinase-1 ratio in acute asthma. *J Allergy Clin Immunol 105*, 900-5.

[92] Galis, Z.S., Sukhova, G.K., Kranzhofer, R., Clark, S., Libby, P. (1995) Macrophage foam cells from experimental atheroma constitutively produce matrix-degrading proteinases. *Proc Natl Acad Sci U S A 92*, 402-6.

[93] Romanic, A.M., Madri, J.A. (1994) The induction of 72-kD gelatinase in T cells upon adhesion to endothelial cells is VCAM-1 dependent. *J Cell Biol 125*, 1165-78.

[94] Goetzl, E.J., Banda, M.J., Leppert, D. (1996) Matrix metalloproteinases in immunity. *J Immunol 156*, 1-4.

[95] John, A., Tuszynski, G. (2001) The role of matrix metalloproteinases in tumor angiogenesis and tumor metastasis. *Pathol Oncol Res 7*, 14-23.

[96] Wagenaar-Miller, R.A., Gorden, L., Matrisian, L.M. (2004) Matrix metalloproteinases in colorectal cancer: is it worth talking about? *Cancer Metastasis Rev 23*, 119-35.

[97] Cross, A.S., Kelly, N.M. (1990) Bacteria-phagocyte interactions: emerging tactics in an ancient rivalry. *FEMS Microbiol Immunol 2*, 245-58.

[98] Babior, B.M. (1999) NADPH oxidase: an update. *Blood 93*, 1464-76.

[99] Klebanoff, S.J. (1980) Oxygen metabolism and the toxic properties of phagocytes. *Ann Intern Med 93*, 480-9.

[100] Rossi, F., Della Bianca, V., de Togni, P. (1985) Mechanisms and functions of the oxygen radicals producing respiration of phagocytes. *Comp Immunol Microbiol Infect Dis 8*, 187-204.

[101] Shepherd, V.L., Hoidal, J.R. (1990) Clearance of neutrophil-derived myeloperoxidase by the macrophage mannose receptor. *Am J Respir Cell Mol Biol 2*, 335-40.

[102] Lincoln, J.A., Lefkowitz, D.L., Cain, T., Castro, A., Mills, K.C., Lefkowitz, S.S., Moguilevsky, N., Bollen, A. (1995) Exogenous myeloperoxidase enhances bacterial phagocytosis and intracellular killing by macrophages. *Infect Immun 63*, 3042-7.

[103] Zgliczynski, J.M., Stelmaszynska, T. (1975) Chlorinating ability of human phagocytosing leucocytes. *Eur J Biochem 56*, 157-62.

[104] Marcinkiewicz, J. (1997) Neutrophil chloramines: missing links between innate and acquired immunity. *Immunol Today 18*, 577-80.

[105] Olszanecki, R., Marcinkiewicz, J. (2004) Taurine chloramine and taurine bromamine induce heme oxygenase-1 in resting and LPS-stimulated J774.2 macrophages. *Amino Acids 27*, 29-35.

[106] Stuehr, D.J., Kwon, N.S., Gross, S.S., Thiel, B.A., Levi, R., Nathan, C.F. (1989) Synthesis of nitrogen oxides from L-arginine by macrophage cytosol: requirement for inducible and constitutive components. *Biochem Biophys Res Commun 161*, 420-6.

[107] Mariotto, S., Menegazzi, M., Suzuki, H. (2004) Biochemical aspects of nitric oxide. *Curr Pharm Des 10*, 1627-45.

[108] Zamora, R., Vodovotz, Y., Billiar, T.R. (2000) Inducible nitric oxide synthase and inflammatory diseases. *Mol Med 6*, 347-73.

[109] McKenna, S.M., Davies, K.J. (1988) Bacterial killing by phagocytes: potential role(s) of hypochlorous acid and hydrogen peroxide in protein turnover, DNA synthesis, and RNA synthesis. *Basic Life Sci 49*, 829-32.

[110] Miyasaki, K.T., Bodeau, A.L. (1991) In vitro killing of Actinobacillus actinomycetemcomitans and Capnocytophaga spp. by human neutrophil cathepsin G and elastase. *Infect Immun 59*, 3015-20.

[111] Ibrahim, H.R., Aoki, T., Pellegrini, A. (2002) Strategies for new antimicrobial proteins and peptides: lysozyme and aprotinin as model molecules. *Curr Pharm Des 8*, 671-93.

[112] Marra, M.N., Wilde, C.G., Collins, M.S., Snable, J.L., Thornton, M.B., Scott, R.W. (1992) The role of bactericidal/permeability-increasing protein as a natural inhibitor of bacterial endotoxin. *J Immunol 148*, 532-7.

[113] Molloy, A.L., Winterbourn, C.C. (1990) Release of iron from phagocytosed Escherichia coli and uptake by neutrophil lactoferrin. *Blood 75*, 984-9.

[114] Diamond, G., Bevins, C.L. (1998) beta-Defensins: endogenous antibiotics of the innate host defense response. *Clin Immunol Immunopathol 88*, 221-5.

[115] Vora, P., Youdim, A., Thomas, L.S., Fukata, M., Tesfay, S.Y., Lukasek, K., Michelsen, K.S., Wada, A., Hirayama, T., Arditi, M., Abreu, M.T. (2004) beta-defensin-2 expression is regulated by TLR signaling in intestinal epithelial cells. *J Immunol 173*, 5398-405.

[116] Lehrer, R.I., Ganz, T. (1990) Antimicrobial polypeptides of human neutrophils. *Blood 76*, 2169-81.

[117] Eaton, J.W. (1993) Defenses against hypochlorous acid: parrying the neutrophil's rapier thrust. *J Lab Clin Med 121*, 197-8.

[118] Koj, A. (1998) Termination of acute-phase response: role of some cytokines and anti-inflammatory drugs. *Gen Pharmacol 31*, 9-18.

[119] Dinarello, C.A. (1997) Role of pro- and anti-inflammatory cytokines during inflammation: experimental and clinical findings. *J Biol Regul Homeost Agents 11*, 91-103.

[120] Gilroy, D.W., Lawrence, T., Perretti, M., Rossi, A.G. (2004) Inflammatory resolution: new opportunities for drug discovery. *Nat Rev Drug Discov 3*, 401-16.

[121] Flower, R.J., Rothwell, N.J. (1994) Lipocortin-1: cellular mechanisms and clinical relevance. *Trends Pharmacol Sci 15*, 71-6.

[122] Perretti, M., Flower, R.J. (2004) Annexin 1 and the biology of the neutrophil. *J Leukoc Biol 76*, 25-9.

[123] Perretti, M., Solito, E. (2004) Annexin 1 and neutrophil apoptosis. *Biochem Soc Trans 32*, 507-10.

[124] Mancuso, F., Flower, R.J., Perretti, M. (1995) Leukocyte transmigration, but not rolling or adhesion, is selectively inhibited by dexamethasone in the hamster post-capillary venule. Involvement of endogenous lipocortin 1. *J Immunol 155*, 377-86.

[125] Adcock, I.M., Ito, K. (2000) Molecular mechanisms of corticosteroid actions. *Monaldi Arch Chest Dis 55*, 256-66.

[126] Wanidworanun, C., Strober, W. (1993) Predominant role of tumor necrosis factor-alpha in human monocyte IL-10 synthesis. *J Immunol 151*, 6853-61.

[127] Guzdek, A., Stalinska, K., Guzik, K., Koj, A. (2000) Differential responses of hematopoietic and non-hematopoietic cells to anti-inflammatory cytokines: IL-4, IL-13 and IL-10. *J Physiol Pharmacol 51*, 387-99.

[128] Capsoni, F., Minonzio, F., Ongari, A.M., Carbonelli, V., Galli, A., Zanussi, C. (1997) Interleukin-10 down-regulates oxidative metabolism and antibody-dependent cellular cytotoxicity of human neutrophils. *Scand J Immunol 45*, 269-75.

[129] Joyce, D.A., Gibbons, D.P., Green, P., Steer, J.H., Feldmann, M., Brennan, F.M. (1994) Two inhibitors of pro-inflammatory cytokine release, interleukin-10 and interleukin-4, have contrasting effects on release of soluble p75 tumor necrosis factor receptor by cultured monocytes. *Eur J Immunol 24*, 2699-705.

[130] Marie, C., Pitton, C., Fitting, C., Cavaillon, J.M. (1996) IL-10 and IL-4 synergize with TNF-alpha to induce IL-1ra production by human neutrophils. *Cytokine 8*, 147-51.

[131] Dinarello, C.A. (2004) Therapeutic strategies to reduce IL-1 activity in treating local and systemic inflammation. *Curr Opin Pharmacol 4*, 378-85.

[132] Dinarello, C.A. (2000) Targeting interleukin 18 with interleukin 18 binding protein. *Ann Rheum Dis 59 Suppl 1*, i17-20.

[133] Aderka, D. (1996) The potential biological and clinical significance of the soluble tumor necrosis factor receptors. *Cytokine Growth Factor Rev 7*, 231-40.

[134] Fernandez-Botran, R., Chilton, P.M., Ma, Y. (1996) Soluble cytokine receptors: their roles in immunoregulation, disease, and therapy. *Adv Immunol 63*, 269-336.

[135] Cichy, J., Rose-John, S., Pryjma, J., Travis, J. (1996) Effect of soluble interleukin-6 receptor on interleukin-6 synthesis in human skin fibroblasts. *Biochem Biophys Res Commun 227*, 318-21.

[136] Kishimoto, T.K., Kahn, J., Migaki, G., Mainolfi, E., Shirley, F., Ingraham, R., Rothlein, R. (1995) Regulation of L-selectin expression by membrane proximal proteolysis. *Agents Actions Suppl 47*, 121-34.

[137] Jones, S.A., Rose-John, S. (2002) The role of soluble receptors in cytokine biology: the agonistic properties of the sIL-6R/IL-6 complex. *Biochim Biophys Acta 1592*, 251-63.

[138] Wertheim, W.A., Kunkel, S.L., Standiford, T.J., Burdick, M.D., Becker, F.S., Wilke, C.A., Gilbert, A.R., Strieter, R.M. (1993) Regulation of neutrophil-derived IL-8: the role of prostaglandin E2, dexamethasone, and IL-4. *J Immunol 151*, 2166-75.

[139] Kasama, T., Strieter, R.M., Lukacs, N.W., Burdick, M.D., Kunkel, S.L. (1994) Regulation of neutrophil-derived chemokine expression by IL-10. *J Immunol 152*, 3559-69.

[140] Sylvester, I., Suffredini, A.F., Boujoukos, A.J., Martich, G.D., Danner, R.L., Yoshimura, T., Leonard, E.J. (1993) Neutrophil attractant protein-1 and monocyte chemoattractant protein-1 in human serum. Effects of intravenous lipopolysaccharide on free attractants, specific IgG autoantibodies and immune complexes. *J Immunol 151*, 3292-8.

[141] Chaudhuri, A., Zbrzezna, V., Polyakova, J., Pogo, A.O., Hesselgesser, J., Horuk, R. (1994) Expression of the Duffy antigen in K562 cells. Evidence that it is the human erythrocyte chemokine receptor. *J Biol Chem 269*, 7835-8.

[142] Luscinskas, F.W., Kiely, J.M., Ding, H., Obin, M.S., Hebert, C.A., Baker, J.B., Gimbrone, M.A., Jr. (1992) In vitro inhibitory effect of IL-8 and other chemoattractants on neutrophil-endothelial adhesive interactions. *J Immunol 149*, 2163-71.

[143] Galli, S.J., Maurer, M., Lantz, C.S. (1999) Mast cells as sentinels of innate immunity. *Curr Opin Immunol 11*, 53-9.

[144] Marshall, J.S., Jawdat, D.M. (2004) Mast cells in innate immunity. *J Allergy Clin Immunol 114*, 21-7.

[145] Galli, S.J. (1993) New concepts about the mast cell. *N Engl J Med 328*, 257-65.

[146] Mekori, Y.A., Metcalfe, D.D. (2000) Mast cells in innate immunity. *Immunol Rev 173*, 131-40.

[147] Schwartz, L.B. (1994) Mast cells: function and contents. *Curr Opin Immunol 6*, 91-7.

[148] Fiorucci, L., Ascoli, F. (2004) Mast cell tryptase, a still enigmatic enzyme. *Cell Mol Life Sci 61*, 1278-95.

[149] Artuc, M., Hermes, B., Steckelings, U.M., Grutzkau, A., Henz, B.M. (1999) Mast cells and their mediators in cutaneous wound healing--active participants or innocent bystanders? *Exp Dermatol 8*, 1-16.

[150] Galli, S.J. (2000) Mast cells and basophils. *Curr Opin Hematol 7*, 32-9.

[151] Abraham, S.N., Arock, M. (1998) Mast cells and basophils in innate immunity. *Semin Immunol 10*, 373-81.

[152] Chuang, W.L., Christ, M.D., Peng, J., Rabenstein, D.L. (2000) An NMR and molecular modeling study of the site-specific binding of histamine by heparin, chemically modified heparin, and heparin-derived oligosaccharides. *Biochemistry 39*, 3542-55.

[153] Prussin, C., Metcalfe, D.D. (2003) 4. IgE, mast cells, basophils, and eosinophils. *J Allergy Clin Immunol 111*, S486-94.

[154] Kinet, J.P. (1989) The high-affinity receptor for IgE. *Curr Opin Immunol 2*, 499-505.

[155] Beaven, M.A., Metzger, H. (1993) Signal transduction by Fc receptors: the Fc epsilon RI case. *Immunol Today 14*, 222-6.

[156] Alber, G., Kent, U.M., Metzger, H. (1992) Functional comparison of Fc epsilon RI, Fc gamma RII, and Fc gamma RIII in mast cells. *J Immunol 149*, 2428-36.

[157] Fruhman, G.J. (1972) The effects of zymosan upon the mast cell population of the peritoneal fluid. *Proc Soc Exp Biol Med 141*, 101-5.

[158] Czarnetzki, B.M. (1982) Release of mediators from purified rat mast cells during phagocytosis. *Scand J Immunol 15*, 581-6.

[159] Leal-Berumen, I., Conlon, P., Marshall, J.S. (1994) IL-6 production by rat peritoneal mast cells is not necessarily preceded by histamine release and can be induced by bacterial lipopolysaccharide. *J Immunol 152*, 5468-76.

[160] Prodeus, A.P., Zhou, X., Maurer, M., Galli, S.J., Carroll, M.C. (1997) Impaired mast cell-dependent natural immunity in complement C3-deficient mice. *Nature 390*, 172-5.

[161] Wojtecka-Lukasik, E., Maslinski, S. (1992) Fibronectin and fibrinogen degradation products stimulate PMN-leukocyte and mast cell degranulation. *J Physiol Pharmacol 43*, 173-81.

[162] Alam, R., Kumar, D., Anderson-Walters, D., Forsythe, P.A. (1994) Macrophage inflammatory protein-1 alpha and monocyte chemoattractant peptide-1 elicit immediate and late cutaneous reactions and activate murine mast cells in vivo. *J Immunol 152*, 1298-303.

[163] Johnston, B., Burns, A.R., Kubes, P. (1998) A role for mast cells in the development of adjuvant-induced vasculitis and arthritis. *Am J Pathol 152*, 555-63.

[164] Meng, H., Tonnesen, M.G., Marchese, M.J., Clark, R.A., Bahou, W.F., Gruber, B.L. (1995) Mast cells are potent regulators of endothelial cell adhesion molecule ICAM-1 and VCAM-1 expression. *J Cell Physiol 165*, 40-53.

[165] Malaviya, R., Ikeda, T., Ross, E., Abraham, S.N. (1996) Mast cell modulation of neutrophil influx and bacterial clearance at sites of infection through TNF-alpha. *Nature 381*, 77-80.

[166] Poncet, P., Arock, M., David, B. (1999) MHC class II-dependent activation of CD4+ T cell hybridomas by human mast cells through superantigen presentation. *J Leukoc Biol 66*, 105-12.

[167] Malaviya, R., Ross, E.A., MacGregor, J.I., Ikeda, T., Little, J.R., Jakschik, B.A., Abraham, S.N. (1994) Mast cell phagocytosis of FimH-expressing enterobacteria. *J Immunol 152*, 1907-14.

[168] Arock, M., Ross, E., Lai-Kuen, R., Averlant, G., Gao, Z., Abraham, S.N. (1998) Phagocytic and tumor necrosis factor alpha response of human mast cells following exposure to gram-negative and gram-positive bacteria. *Infect Immun 66*, 6030-4.

[169] Rodewald, H.R., Dessing, M., Dvorak, A.M., Galli, S.J. (1996) Identification of a committed precursor for the mast cell lineage. *Science 271*, 818-22.

[170] Kirshenbaum, A.S., Goff, J.P., Semere, T., Foster, B., Scott, L.M., Metcalfe, D.D. (1999) Demonstration that human mast cells arise from a progenitor cell population that is CD34(+), c-kit(+), and expresses aminopeptidase N (CD13). *Blood 94*, 2333-42.

[171] Kitamura, Y., Go, S. (1979) Decreased production of mast cells in S1/S1d anemic mice. *Blood 53*, 492-7.

[172] Sonoda, T., Ohno, T., Kitamura, Y. (1982) Concentration of mast-cell progenitors in bone marrow, spleen, and blood of mice determined by limiting dilution analysis. *J Cell Physiol 112*, 136-40.

[173] Kobayashi, T., Nakano, T., Nakahata, T., Asai, H., Yagi, Y., Tsuji, K., Komiyama, A., Akabane, T., Kojima, S., Kitamura, Y. (1986) Formation of mast cell colonies in methylcellulose by mouse peritoneal cells and differentiation of these cloned cells in both the skin and the gastric mucosa of W/Wv mice: evidence that a common precursor can give rise to both "connective tissue-type" and "mucosal" mast cells. *J Immunol 136*, 1378-84.

[174] Bienenstock, J., Befus, A.D., Pearce, F., Denburg, J., Goodacre, R. (1982) Mast cell heterogeneity: derivation and function, with emphasis on the intestine. *J Allergy Clin Immunol 70*, 407-12.

[175] Yecies, L.D., Johnson, S.M., Wedner, H.J., Parker, C.W. (1979) Slow reacting substance (SRS) from ionophore A23187-stimulated peritoneal mast cells of the normal rat. II. Evidence for a precursor role of arachidonic acid and further purification. *J Immunol 122*, 2090-5.

[176] Razin, E., Stevens, R.L., Akiyama, F., Schmid, K., Austen, K.F. (1982) Culture from mouse bone marrow of a subclass of mast cells possessing a distinct chondroitin sulfate proteoglycan with glycosaminoglycans rich in N-acetylgalactosamine-4,6-disulfate. *J Biol Chem 257*, 7229-36.

[177] Razin, E., Mencia-Huerta, J.M., Lewis, R.A., Corey, E.J., Austen, K.F. (1982) Generation of leukotriene C4 from a subclass of mast cells differentiated in vitro from mouse bone marrow. *Proc Natl Acad Sci U S A 79*, 4665-7.

[178] Lantz, C.S., Boesiger, J., Song, C.H., Mach, N., Kobayashi, T., Mulligan, R.C., Nawa, Y., Dranoff, G., Galli, S.J. (1998) Role for interleukin-3 in mast-cell and basophil development and in immunity to parasites. *Nature 392*, 90-3.

[179] Liu, H., Pope, R.M. (2004) Phagocytes: mechanisms of inflammation and tissue destruction. *Rheum Dis Clin North Am 30*, 19-39, v.

[180] Naito, M., Hasegawa, G., Ebe, Y., Yamamoto, T. (2004) Differentiation and function of Kupffer cells. *Med Electron Microsc 37*, 16-28.

[181] Rutherford, M.S., Witsell, A., Schook, L.B. (1993) Mechanisms generating functionally heterogeneous macrophages: chaos revisited. *J Leukoc Biol 53*, 602-18.

[182] Morrissette, N., Gold, E., Aderem, A. (1999) The macrophage--a cell for all seasons. *Trends Cell Biol 9*, 199-201.

[183] Borrello, M.A., Phipps, R.P. (1996) The B/macrophage cell: an elusive link between CD5+ B lymphocytes and macrophages. *Immunol Today 17*, 471-5.

[184] Phipps, R.P., Pollock, S.J., Kaur, K., Kaufman, J., Borrello, M.A., Graf, B.A., Nazarenko, D., Roberts, L.J., Morrow, J.D., Palis, J., Ryan, D.J., Bennett, J.M. (2000) Expression of cyclooxygenase-2 and prostaglandins by B-1 cells and B-CLL cells. *Curr Top Microbiol Immunol 252*, 293-300.

[185] Graf, B.A., Nazarenko, D.A., Borrello, M.A., Roberts, L.J., Morrow, J.D., Palis, J., Phipps, R.P. (1999) Biphenotypic B/macrophage cells express COX-1 and up-regulate COX-2 expression and prostaglandin E(2) production in response to pro-inflammatory signals. *Eur J Immunol 29*, 3793-803.

[186] Plytycz, B., Seljelid, R. (1997) B-1/macrophages as 'living fossils'. *Immunol Today 18*, 505.

[187] Wake, K., Kawai, Y., Smedsrod, B. (2001) Re-evaluation of the reticulo-endothelial system. *Ital J Anat Embryol 106*, 261-9.

[188] Smedsrod, B., Pertoft, H., Gustafson, S., Laurent, T.C. (1990) Scavenger functions of the liver endothelial cell. *Biochem J 266*, 313-27.

[189] Smedsrod, B., De Bleser, P.J., Braet, F., Lovisetti, P., Vanderkerken, K., Wisse, E., Geerts, A. (1994) Cell biology of liver endothelial and Kupffer cells. *Gut 35*, 1509-16.

[190] Rabinovitch, M. (1995) Professional and non-professional phagocytes: an introduction. *Trends Cell Biol 5*, 85-7.

[191] Stahl, P.D., Ezekowitz, R.A. (1998) The mannose receptor is a pattern recognition receptor involved in host defense. *Curr Opin Immunol 10*, 50-5.

[192] van der Laan, L.J., Dopp, E.A., Haworth, R., Pikkarainen, T., Kangas, M., Elomaa, O., Dijkstra, C.D., Gordon, S., Tryggvason, K., Kraal, G. (1999) Regulation and functional involvement of macrophage scavenger receptor MARCO in clearance of bacteria in vivo. *J Immunol 162*, 939-47.

[193] Platt, N., Haworth, R., Darley, L., Gordon, S. (2002) The many roles of the class A macrophage scavenger receptor. *Int Rev Cytol 212*, 1-40.

[194] Ravetch, J.V., Clynes, R.A. (1998) Divergent roles for Fc receptors and complement in vivo. *Annu Rev Immunol 16*, 421-32.

[195] Aderem, A., Underhill, D.M. (1999) Mechanisms of phagocytosis in macrophages. *Annu Rev Immunol 17*, 593-623.

[196] Keshav, S., Chung, L.P., Gordon, S. (1990) Macrophage products in inflammation. *Diagn Microbiol Infect Dis 13*, 439-47.

[197] Grage-Griebenow, E., Flad, H.D., Ernst, M., Bzowska, M., Skrzeczynska, J., Pryjma, J. (2000) Human MO subsets as defined by expression of CD64 and CD16 differ in phagocytic activity and generation of oxygen intermediates. *Immunobiology 202*, 42-50.

[198] Nathan, C.F. (1987) Secretory products of macrophages. *J Clin Invest 79*, 319-26.

[199] Underhill, D.M., Ozinsky, A., Hajjar, A.M., Stevens, A., Wilson, C.B., Bassetti, M., Aderem, A. (1999) The Toll-like receptor 2 is recruited to macrophage phagosomes and discriminates between pathogens. *Nature 401*, 811-5.

[200] Gregory, C.D., Devitt, A. (2004) The macrophage and the apoptotic cell: an innate immune interaction viewed simplistically? *Immunology 113*, 1-14.

[201] Adams, D.O., Hamilton, T.A. (1987) Molecular transductional mechanisms by which IFN gamma and other signals regulate macrophage development. *Immunol Rev 97*, 5-27.

[202] Belosevic, M., Davis, C.E., Meltzer, M.S., Nacy, C.A. (1988) Regulation of activated macrophage antimicrobial activities. Identification of lymphokines that cooperate with IFN-gamma for induction of resistance to infection. *J Immunol 141*, 890-6.

[203] van Rooijen, N., Wijburg, O.L., van den Dobbelsteen, G.P., Sanders, A. (1996) Macrophages in host defense mechanisms. *Curr Top Microbiol Immunol 210*, 159-65.

[204] Baran, J., Pryjma, J. (1994) The reduced expression of HLA-class II antigens and adhesion molecules on monocyte surface after phagocytosis of bacteria. *Arch Immunol Ther Exp (Warsz) 42*, 101-6.

[205] Pryjma, J., Baran, J., Ernst, M., Woloszyn, M., Flad, H.D. (1994) Altered antigen-presenting capacity of human monocytes after phagocytosis of bacteria. *Infect Immun 62*, 1961-7.

[206] Baran, J., Guzik, K., Hryniewicz, W., Ernst, M., Flad, H.D., Pryjma, J. (1996) Apoptosis of monocytes and prolonged survival of granulocytes as a result of phagocytosis of bacteria. *Infect Immun 64*, 4242-8.

[207] Flad, H.D., Grage-Griebenow, E., Petersen, F., Scheuerer, B., Brandt, E., Baran, J., Pryjma, J., Ernst, M. (1999) The role of cytokines in monocyte apoptosis. *Pathobiology 67*, 291-3.

[208] Becker, E.L. (1990) The short and happy life of neutrophil activation. *J Leukoc Biol 47*, 378-89.

[209] Boggs, D.R. (1967) The kinetics of neutrophilic leukocytes in health and in disease. *Semin Hematol 4*, 359-86.

[210] Ratcliffe, D.R., Nolin, S.L., Cramer, E.B. (1988) Neutrophil interaction with influenza-infected epithelial cells. *Blood 72*, 142-9.

[211] Weiss, S.J. (1989) Tissue destruction by neutrophils. *N Engl J Med 320*, 365-76.

[212] Borregaard, N., Lollike, K., Kjeldsen, L., Sengelov, H., Bastholm, L., Nielsen, M.H., Bainton, D.F. (1993) Human neutrophil granules and secretory vesicles. *Eur J Haematol 51*, 187-98.

[213] Quinn, M.T., Gauss, K.A. (2004) Structure and regulation of the neutrophil respiratory burst oxidase: comparison with nonphagocyte oxidases. *J Leukoc Biol 76*, 760-81.

[214] Grage-Griebenow, E., Durrbaum-Landmann, I., Pryjma, J., Loppnow, H., Flad, H.D., Ernst, M. (1998) Apoptosis in monocytes. *Eur Cytokine Netw 9*, 699-700.

[215] Fadeel, B., Ahlin, A., Henter, J.I., Orrenius, S., Hampton, M.B. (1998) Involvement of caspases in neutrophil apoptosis: regulation by reactive oxygen species. *Blood 92*, 4808-18.

[216] Savill, J., Fadok, V., Henson, P., Haslett, C. (1993) Phagocyte recognition of cells undergoing apoptosis. *Immunol Today 14*, 131-6.

[217] Murray, J., Barbara, J.A., Dunkley, S.A., Lopez, A.F., Van Ostade, X., Condliffe, A.M., Dransfield, I., Haslett, C., Chilvers, E.R. (1997) Regulation of neutrophil apoptosis by tumor necrosis factor-alpha: requirement for TNFR55 and TNFR75 for induction of apoptosis *in vitro*. *Blood 90*, 2772-83.

[218] Denkers, E.Y., Del Rio, L., Bennouna, S. (2003) Neutrophil production of IL-12 and other cytokines during microbial infection. *Chem Immunol Allergy 83*, 95-114.

[219] Fujishima, S., Hoffman, A.R., Vu, T., Kim, K.J., Zheng, H., Daniel, D., Kim, Y., Wallace, E.F., Larrick, J.W., Raffin, T.A. (1993) Regulation of neutrophil interleukin 8 gene expression and protein secretion by LPS, TNF-alpha, and IL-1 beta. *J Cell Physiol 154*, 478-85.

[220] Kasama, T., Strieter, R.M., Standiford, T.J., Burdick, M.D., Kunkel, S.L. (1993) Expression and regulation of human neutrophil-derived macrophage inflammatory protein 1 alpha. *J Exp Med 178*, 63-72.

[221] Ajuebor, M.N., Flower, R.J., Hannon, R., Christie, M., Bowers, K., Verity, A., Perretti, M. (1998) Endogenous monocyte chemoattractant protein-1 recruits monocytes in the zymosan peritonitis model. *J Leukoc Biol 63*, 108-16.

[222] Terebuh, P.D., Otterness, I.G., Strieter, R.M., Lincoln, P.M., Danforth, J.M., Kunkel, S.L., Chensue, S.W. (1992) Biologic and immunohistochemical analysis of interleukin-6 expression in vivo. Constitutive and induced expression in murine polymorphonuclear and mononuclear phagocytes. *Am J Pathol 140*, 649-57.

[223] Matsukawa, A., Yoshinaga, M. (1999) Neutrophils as a source of cytokines in inflammation. *Histol Histopathol 14*, 511-6.

[224] Schroder, J.M. (1992) The neutrophil-activating peptide 1/interleukin 8, a novel neutrophil chemotactic cytokine. *Arch Immunol Ther Exp (Warsz) 40*, 23-31.

[225] Sala, A., Folco, G. (2001) Neutrophils, endothelial cells, and cysteinyl leukotrienes: a new approach to neutrophil-dependent inflammation? *Biochem Biophys Res Commun 283*, 1003-6.

[226] Vercellotti, G.M., Yin, H.Q., Gustafson, K.S., Nelson, R.D., Jacob, H.S. (1988) Platelet-activating factor primes neutrophil responses to agonists: role in promoting neutrophil-mediated endothelial damage. *Blood 71*, 1100-7.

[227] Malaviya, R., Abraham, S.N. (2000) Role of mast cell leukotrienes in neutrophil recruitment and bacterial clearance in infectious peritonitis. *J Leukoc Biol 67*, 841-6.

[228] Marcinkiewicz, J. (2003) Prostanoids and MPO-halide system products as a link between innate and adaptive immunity. *Immunol Lett 89*, 187-91.

[229] Spector, W.G. (1958) Substances which affect capillary permeability. *Pharmacol Rev 10*, 475-505.

[230] Movat, H.Z. (1987) The role of histamine and other mediators in microvascular changes in acute inflammation. *Can J Physiol Pharmacol 65*, 451-7.

[231] Riley, J.F., West, G.B. (1966) The occurance of histamine in mast cells. In *Handbook of Experimental Pharmacology*, Volume 18, part 1 (M. Rocha and E. Silva, eds), Springer-Verlag, Berlin 116-135.

[232] MacGlashan, D., Jr. (2003) Histamine: A mediator of inflammation. *J Allergy Clin Immunol 112*, S53 9.

[233] Sampson, D., Archer, G.T. (1967) Release of histamine from human basophils. *Blood 29*, 722-36.

[234] Saxena, S.P., McNicol, A., Brandes, L.J., Becker, A.B., Gerrard, J.M. (1989) Histamine formed in stimulated human platelets is cytoplasmic. *Biochem Biophys Res Commun 164*, 164-8.

[235] El-Ackad, T.M., Brody, M.J. (1975) Evidence for non-mast cell histamine in the vascular wall. *Blood Vessels 12*, 181-91.

[236] Karnushina, I.L., Palacios, J.M., Barbin, G., Dux, E., Joo, F., Schwartz, J.C. (1980) Studies on a capillary-rich fraction isolated from brain: histaminic components and characterization of the histamine receptors linked to adenylate cyclase. *J Neurochem 34*, 1201-8.

[237] Schwartz, J.C., Pollard, H., Quach, T.T. (1980) Histamine as a neurotransmitter in mammalian brain: neurochemical evidence. *J Neurochem 35*, 26-33.

[238] Lewis, G.P., Mangham, B.A. (1978) Changes in blood flow, histamine and prostaglandin E2 in rabbit skin grafts [proceedings]. *Br J Pharmacol 62*, 420P-421P.

[239] Hill, S.J. (1990) Distribution, properties, and functional characteristics of three classes of histamine receptor. *Pharmacol Rev 42*, 45-83.

[240] Wardlaw, A.C., Parton, R., Hooker, M.J. (1976) Loss of protective antigen, histamine-sensitising factor and envelope polypeptides in cultural variants of Bordetella pertussis. *J Med Microbiol 9*, 89-100.

[241] Kroeze, W.K., Kristiansen, K., Roth, B.L. (2002) Molecular biology of serotonin receptors structure and function at the molecular level. *Curr Top Med Chem 2*, 507-28.

[242] Mitsuhashi, M., Payan, D.G. (1992) Functional diversity of histamine and histamine receptors. *J Invest Dermatol 98*, 8S-11S.

[243] Cameron, W., Doyle, K., Rocklin, R.E. (1986) Histamine type I (H1) receptor radioligand binding studies on normal T cell subsets, B cells, and monocytes. *J Immunol 136*, 2116-20.

[244] Falus, A. (1994) Histamine modulates the acute phase response at multiple points. *Immunol Today 15*, 596.

[245] Hellstrand, K., Asea, A., Hermodsson, S. (1990) Role of histamine in natural killer cell-mediated resistance against tumor cells. *J Immunol 145*, 4365-70.

[246] Seligmann, B.E., Fletcher, M.P., Gallin, J.I. (1983) Histamine modulation of human neutrophil oxidative metabolism, locomotion, degranulation, and membrane potential changes. *J Immunol 130*, 1902-9.

[247] Dohlsten, M., Sjogren, H.O., Carlsson, R. (1987) Histamine acts directly on human T cells to inhibit interleukin-2 and interferon-gamma production. *Cell Immunol 109*, 65-74.

[248] Vannier, E., Miller, L.C., Dinarello, C.A. (1991) Histamine suppresses gene expression and synthesis of tumor necrosis factor alpha via histamine H2 receptors. *J Exp Med 174*, 281-4.

[249] Tung, R., Kagey-Sobotka, A., Plaut, M., Lichtenstein, L.M. (1982) H2 antihistamines augment antigen-induced histamine release from human basophils in vitro. *J Immunol 129*, 2113-5.

[250] Melmon, K.L., Bourne, H.R., Weinstein, Y., Shearer, G.M., Kram, J., Bauminger, S. (1974) Hemolytic plaque formation by leukocytes in vitro. Control by vasoactive hormones. *J Clin Invest 53*, 13-21.

[251] Melmon, K.L., Rocklin, R.E., Rosenkranz, R.P. (1981) Autacoids as modulators of the inflammatory and immune response. *Am J Med 71*, 100-6.

[252] Hill, S.J., Ganellin, C.R., Timmerman, H., Schwartz, J.C., Shankley, N.P., Young, J.M., Schunack, W., Levi, R., Haas, H.L. (1997) International Union of Pharmacology. XIII. Classification of histamine receptors. *Pharmacol Rev 49*, 253-78.

[253] Bakker, R.A., Timmerman, H., Leurs, R. (2002) Histamine receptors: specific ligands, receptor biochemistry, and signal transduction. *Clin Allergy Immunol 17*, 27-64.

[254] Hough, L.B. (2001) Genomics meets histamine receptors: new subtypes, new receptors. *Mol Pharmacol 59*, 415-9.

[255] Timmerman, H. (1992) Cloning of the H1 histamine receptor. *Trends Pharmacol Sci 13*, 6-7.

[256] Marceau, F., Regoli, D. (2004) Bradykinin receptor ligands: therapeutic perspectives. *Nat Rev Drug Discov 3*, 845-52.

[257] Reissmann, S., Pineda, F., Vietinghoff, G., Werner, H., Gera, L., Stewart, J.M., Paegelow, I. (2000) Structure activity relationships for bradykinin antagonists on the inhibition of cytokine release and the release of histamine. *Peptides 21*, 527-33.

[258] Said, S.I. (1983) Vasoactive peptides. State-of-the-art review. *Hypertension 5*, I17-26.

[259] Datar, P., Srivastava, S., Coutinho, E., Govil, G. (2004) Substance P: structure, function, and therapeutics. *Curr Top Med Chem 4*, 75-103.

[260] Ceciliani, F., Giordano, A., Spagnolo, V. (2002) The systemic reaction during inflammation: the acute-phase proteins. *Protein Pept Lett 9*, 211-23.

[261] Cunnane, G., Whitehead, A.S. (1999) Amyloid precursors and amyloidosis in rheumatoid arthritis. *Baillieres Best Pract Res Clin Rheumatol 13*, 615-28.

[262] Mortensen, R.F., Zhong, W. (2000) Regulation of phagocytic leukocyte activities by C-reactive protein. *J Leukoc Biol 67*, 495-500.

[263] Du Clos, T.W. (2000) Function of C-reactive protein. *Ann Med 32*, 274-8.

[264] Uhlar, C.M., Whitehead, A.S. (1999) Serum amyloid A, the major vertebrate acute-phase reactant. *Eur J Biochem 265*, 501-23.

[265] Urieli-Shoval, S., Linke, R.P., Matzner, Y. (2000) Expression and function of serum amyloid A, a major acute-phase protein, in normal and disease states. *Curr Opin Hematol 7*, 64-9.

[266] Wang, Y., Ripperger, J., Fey, G.H., Samols, D., Kordula, T., Wetzler, M., Van Etten, R.A., Baumann, H. (1999) Modulation of hepatic acute phase gene expression by epidermal growth factor and Src protein tyrosine kinases in murine and human hepatic cells. *Hepatology 30*, 682-97.

[267] Santoro, M.G. (2000) Heat shock factors and the control of the stress response. *Biochem Pharmacol 59*, 55-63.

[268] Feder, M.E., Hofmann, G.E. (1999) Heat-shock proteins, molecular chaperones, and the stress response: evolutionary and ecological physiology. *Annu Rev Physiol 61*, 243-82.

[269] Lindquist, S., Craig, E.A. (1988) The heat-shock proteins. *Annu Rev Genet 22*, 631-77.

[270] Feige, U., van Eden, W. (1996) Infection, autoimmunity and autoimmune disease. *Exs 77*, 359-73.

[271] Malhotra, V., Wong, H.R. (2002) Interactions between the heat shock response and the nuclear factor-kappaB signaling pathway. *Crit Care Med 30*, S89-S95.

[272] Wong, H.R. (1998) Potential protective role of the heat shock response in sepsis. *New Horiz 6*, 194-200.

[273] Kim, H.D., Kang, H.S., Rimbach, G., Park, Y.C. (1999) Heat shock and 5-azacytidine inhibit nitric oxide synthesis and tumor necrosis factor-alpha secretion in activated macrophages. *Antioxid Redox Signal 1*, 297-304.

[274] Barnes, P.J. (1997) Nuclear factor-kappa B. *Int J Biochem Cell Biol 29*, 867-70.

[275] Narumiya, S. (2003) Prostanoids in immunity: roles revealed by mice deficient in their receptors. *Life Sci 74*, 391-5.

[276] Clissold, D., Thickitt, C. (1994) Recent eicosanoid chemistry. *Nat Prod Rep 11*, 621-37.

[277] Narumiya, S., Sugimoto, Y., Ushikubi, F. (1999) Prostanoid receptors: structures, properties, and functions. *Physiol Rev 79*, 1193-226.

[278] Salmon, J.A., Higgs, G.A. (1987) Prostaglandins and leukotrienes as inflammatory mediators. *Br Med Bull 43*, 285-96.

[279] Bulger, E.M., Maier, R.V. (2000) Lipid mediators in the pathophysiology of critical illness. *Crit Care Med 28*, N27-36.

[280] Gijon, M.A., Leslie, C.C. (1999) Regulation of arachidonic acid release and cytosolic phospholipase A2 activation. *J Leukoc Biol 65*, 330-6.

[281] Qiu, Z.H., Gijon, M.A., de Carvalho, M.S., Spencer, D.M., Leslie, C.C. (1998) The role of calcium and phosphorylation of cytosolic phospholipase A2 in regulating arachidonic acid release in macrophages. *J Biol Chem 273*, 8203-11.

[282] Serhan, C.N., Haeggstrom, J.Z., Leslie, C.C. (1996) Lipid mediator networks in cell signaling: update and impact of cytokines. *Faseb J 10*, 1147-58.

[283] Peters-Golden, M., Brock, T.G. (2003) 5-lipoxygenase and FLAP. *Prostaglandins Leukot Essent Fatty Acids 69*, 99-109.

[284] Heller, A., Koch, T., Schmeck, J., van Ackern, K. (1998) Lipid mediators in inflammatory disorders. *Drugs 55*, 487-96.

[285] Chen, X.S., Naumann, T.A., Kurre, U., Jenkins, N.A., Copeland, N.G., Funk, C.D. (1995) cDNA cloning, expression, mutagenesis, intracellular localization, and gene chromosomal assignment of mouse 5-lipoxygenase. *J Biol Chem 270*, 17993-9.

[286] Willoughby, D.A., Moore, A.R., Colville-Nash, P.R. (2000) COX-1, COX-2, and COX-3 and the future treatment of chronic inflammatory disease. *Lancet 355*, 646-8.

[287] Warner, T.D., Vojnovic, I., Giuliano, F., Jimenez, R., Bishop-Bailey, D., Mitchell, J.A. (2004) Cyclooxygenases 1, 2, and 3 and the production of prostaglandin i2: investigating the activities of acetaminophen and cyclooxygenase-2-selective inhibitors in rat tissues. *J Pharmacol Exp Ther 310*, 642-7.

[288] Warner, T.D., Mitchell, J.A. (2004) Cyclooxygenases: new forms, new inhibitors, and lessons from the clinic. *Faseb J 18*, 790-804.

[289] Kiefer, J.R., Pawlitz, J.L., Moreland, K.T., Stegeman, R.A., Hood, W.F., Gierse, J.K., Stevens, A.M., Goodwin, D.C., Rowlinson, S.W., Marnett, L.J., Stallings, W.C., Kurumbail, R.G. (2000) Structural insights into the stereochemistry of the cyclooxygenase reaction. *Nature 405*, 97-101.

[290] Reddy, S.T., Herschman, H.R. (1996) Transcellular prostaglandin production following mast cell activation is mediated by proximal secretory phospholipase A2 and distal prostaglandin synthase 1. *J Biol Chem 271*, 186-91.

[291] Dubois, R.N., Abramson, S.B., Crofford, L., Gupta, R.A., Simon, L.S., Van De Putte, L.B., Lipsky, P.E. (1998) Cyclooxygenase in biology and disease. *Faseb J 12*, 1063-73.

[292] Langenbach, R., Loftin, C.D., Lee, C., Tiano, H. (1999) Cyclooxygenase-deficient mice. A summary of their characteristics and susceptibilities to inflammation and carcinogenesis. *Ann N Y Acad Sci 889*, 52-61.

[293] Murakami, M., Kambe, T., Shimbara, S., Kudo, I. (1999) Functional coupling between various phospholipase A2s and cyclooxygenases in immediate and delayed prostanoid biosynthetic pathways. *J Biol Chem 274*, 3103-15.

[294] MacNaughton, W.K., Cushing, K. (2000) Role of constitutive cyclooxygenase-2 in prostaglandin-dependent secretion in mouse colon in vitro. *J Pharmacol Exp Ther 293*, 539-44.

[295] McAdam, B.F., Catella-Lawson, F., Mardini, I.A., Kapoor, S., Lawson, J.A., FitzGerald, G.A. (1999) Systemic biosynthesis of prostacyclin by cyclooxygenase (COX)-2: the human pharmacology of a selective inhibitor of COX-2. *Proc Natl Acad Sci U S A 96*, 272-7.

[296] Yasojima, K., Schwab, C., McGeer, E.G., McGeer, P.L. (1999) Distribution of cyclooxygenase-1 and cyclooxygenase-2 mRNAs and proteins in human brain and peripheral organs. *Brain Res 830*, 226-36.

[297] Jun, S.S., Chen, Z., Pace, M.C., Shaul, P.W. (1998) Estrogen upregulates cyclooxygenase-1 gene expression in ovine fetal pulmonary artery endothelium. *J Clin Invest 102*, 176-83.

[298] Chandrasekharan, N.V., Dai, H., Roos, K.L., Evanson, N.K., Tomsik, J., Elton, T.S., Simmons, D.L. (2002) COX-3, a cyclooxygenase-1 variant inhibited by acetaminophen and other analgesic/antipyretic drugs: cloning, structure, and expression. *Proc Natl Acad Sci U S A 99*, 13926-31.

[299] Chandrasekharan, N.V., Simmons, D.L. (2004) The cyclooxygenases. *Genome Biol 5*, 241.

[300] Werz, O. (2002) 5-lipoxygenase: cellular biology and molecular pharmacology. *Curr Drug Targets Inflamm Allergy 1*, 23-44.

[301] Kobayashi, T., Narumiya, S. (2002) Function of prostanoid receptors: studies on knockout mice. *Prostaglandins Other Lipid Mediat 68-69*, 557-73.

[302] Kanaoka, Y., Boyce, J.A. (2004) Cysteinyl leukotrienes and their receptors: cellular distribution and function in immune and inflammatory responses. *J Immunol 173*, 1503-10.

[303] Hedqvist, P., Gautam, N., Lindbom, L. (2000) Interactions between leukotrienes and other inflammatory mediators/modulators in the microvasculature. *Am J Respir Crit Care Med 161*, S117-9.

[304] Coceani, F., Akarsu, E.S. (1998) Prostaglandin E2 in the pathogenesis of fever. An update. *Ann N Y Acad Sci 856*, 76-82.

[305] Zhang, X.W., Liu, Q., Wang, Y., Thorlacius, H. (2001) CXC chemokines, MIP-2 and KC, induce P-selectin-dependent neutrophil rolling and extravascular migration in vivo. *Br J Pharmacol 133*, 413-21.

[306] Paoletti, S., Petkovic, V., Sebastiani, S., Danelon, M.G., Uguccioni, M., Gerber, B.O. (2004) A rich chemokine environment strongly enhances leukocyte migration and activities. *Bloo, 105,* 3405-12.

[307] Lukacs, N.W., Kunkel, S.L. (1998) Chemokines and their role in disease. *Int J Clin Lab Res 28*, 91-5.

[308] Detmers, P.A., Lo, S.K., Olsen-Egbert, E., Walz, A., Baggiolini, M., Cohn, Z.A. (1990) Neutrophil-activating protein 1/interleukin 8 stimulates the binding activity of the leukocyte adhesion receptor CD11b/CD18 on human neutrophils. *J Exp Med 171*, 1155-62.

[309] Smart, S.J., Casale, T.B. (1994) TNF-alpha-induced transendothelial neutrophil migration is IL-8 dependent. *Am J Physiol 266*, L238-45.

[310] Walz, A., Meloni, F., Clark-Lewis, I., von Tscharner, V., Baggiolini, M. (1991) [Ca2+]i changes and respiratory burst in human neutrophils and monocytes induced by NAP-1/interleukin-8, NAP-2, and gro/MGSA. *J Leukoc Biol 50*, 279-86.

[311] Perretti, M., Harris, J.G., Flower, R.J. (1994) A role for endogenous histamine in interleukin-8-induced neutrophil infiltration into mouse air-pouch: investigation of the modulatory action of systemic and local dexamethasone. *Br J Pharmacol 112*, 801-8.

[312] Alam, R., Forsythe, P., Stafford, S., Heinrich, J., Bravo, R., Proost, P., Van Damme, J. (1994) Monocyte chemotactic protein-2, monocyte chemotactic protein-3, and fibroblast-induced cytokine. Three new chemokines induce chemotaxis and activation of basophils. *J Immunol 153*, 3155-9.

[313] Feghali, C.A., Wright, T.M. (1997) Cytokines in acute and chronic inflammation. *Front Biosci 2*, d12-26.

[314] Goetz, F.W., Planas, J.V., MacKenzie, S. (2004) Tumor necrosis factors. *Dev Comp Immunol 28*, 487-97.

[315] Nawroth, P.P., Bank, I., Handley, D., Cassimeris, J., Chess, L., Stern, D. (1986) Tumor necrosis factor/cachectin interacts with endothelial cell receptors to induce release of interleukin 1. *J Exp Med 163*, 1363-75.

[316] Nawroth, P.P., Handley, D.A., Esmon, C.T., Stern, D.M. (1986) Interleukin 1 induces endothelial cell procoagulant while suppressing cell-surface anticoagulant activity. *Proc Natl Acad Sci U S A 83*, 3460-4.

[317] Vilcek, J., Lee, T.H. (1991) Tumor necrosis factor. New insights into the molecular mechanisms of its multiple actions. *J Biol Chem 266*, 7313-6.

[318] Idriss, H.T., Naismith, J.H. (2000) TNF alpha and the TNF receptor superfamily: structure-function relationship(s). *Microsc Res Tech 50*, 184-95.

[319] Black, R.A., Rauch, C.T., Kozlosky, C.J., Peschon, J.J., Slack, J.L., Wolfson, M.F., Castner, B.J., Stocking, K.L., Reddy, P., Srinivasan, S., Nelson, N., Boiani, N., Schooley, K.A., Gerhart, M., Davis, R., Fitzner, J.N., Johnson, R.S., Paxton, R.J., March, C.J., Cerretti, D.P. (1997) A metalloproteinase disintegrin that releases tumour-necrosis factor-alpha from cells. *Nature 385*, 729-33.

[320] Dinarello, C.A. (2002) The IL-1 family and inflammatory diseases. *Clin Exp Rheumatol 20*, S1-13.

[321] Warren, J.S. (1990) Interleukins and tumor necrosis factor in inflammation. *Crit Rev Clin Lab Sci 28*, 37-59.

[322] Cullinan, E.B., Kwee, L., Nunes, P., Shuster, D.J., Ju, G., McIntyre, K.W., Chizzonite, R.A., Labow, M.A. (1998) IL-1 receptor accessory protein is an essential component of the IL-1 receptor. *J Immunol 161*, 5614-20.

[323] Colotta, F., Dower, S.K., Sims, J.E., Mantovani, A. (1994) The type II 'decoy' receptor: a novel regulatory pathway for interleukin 1. *Immunol Today 15*, 562-6.

[324] Sims, J.E., Giri, J.G., Dower, S.K. (1994) The two interleukin-1 receptors play different roles in IL-1 actions. *Clin Immunol Immunopathol 72*, 9-14.

[325] Dinarello, C.A. (1996) Biologic basis for interleukin-1 in disease. *Blood 87*, 2095-147.

[326] Hacham, M., Argov, S., White, R.M., Segal, S., Apte, R.N. (2000) Distinct patterns of IL-1 alpha and IL-1 beta organ distribution--a possible basis for organ mechanisms of innate immunity. *Adv Exp Med Biol 479*, 185-202.

[327] Thornberry, N.A., Bull, H.G., Calaycay, J.R., Chapman, K.T., Howard, A.D., Kostura, M.J., Miller, D.K., Molineaux, S.M., Weidner, J.R., Aunins, J., et al. (1992) A novel heterodimeric cysteine protease is required for interleukin-1 beta processing in monocytes. *Nature 356*, 768-74.

[328] Dinarello, C.A., Fantuzzi, G. (2003) Interleukin-18 and host defense against infection. *J Infect Dis 187 Suppl 2*, S370-84.

[329] Mencacci, A., Bacci, A., Cenci, E., Montagnoli, C., Fiorucci, S., Casagrande, A., Flavell, R.A., Bistoni, F., Romani, L. (2000) Interleukin 18 restores defective Th1 immunity to Candida albicans in caspase 1-deficient mice. *Infect Immun 68*, 5126-31.

[330] Dinarello, C.A., Novick, D., Rubinstein, M., Lonnemann, G. (2003) Interleukin 18 and interleukin 18 binding protein: possible role in immunosuppression of chronic renal failure. *Blood Purif 21*, 258-70.

[331] Okamura, H., Tsutsi, H., Komatsu, T., Yutsudo, M., Hakura, A., Tanimoto, T., Torigoe, K., Okura, T., Nukada, Y., Hattori, K., et al. (1995) Cloning of a new cytokine that induces IFN-gamma production by T cells. *Nature 378*, 88-91.

[332] Porat, R., Poutsiaka, D.D., Miller, L.C., Granowitz, E.V., Dinarello, C.A. (1992) Interleukin-1 (IL-1) receptor blockade reduces endotoxin and Borrelia burgdorferi-stimulated IL-8 synthesis in human mononuclear cells. *Faseb J 6*, 2482-6.

[333] Angel, J., Audubert, F., Bismuth, G., Fournier, C. (1994) IL-1 beta amplifies bradykinin-induced prostaglandin E2 production via a phospholipase D-linked mechanism. *J Immunol 152*, 5032-40.

[334] Subramanian, N., Bray, M.A. (1987) Interleukin 1 releases histamine from human basophils and mast cells in vitro. *J Immunol 138*, 271-5.

[335] Tilg, H., Dinarello, C.A., Mier, J.W. (1997) IL-6 and APPs: anti-inflammatory and immunosuppressive mediators. *Immunol Today 18*, 428-32.

[336] Dantzer, R. (2001) Cytokine-induced sickness behavior: where do we stand? *Brain Behav Immun 15*, 7-24.

[337] van Dam, A.M., Brouns, M., Louisse, S., Berkenbosch, F. (1992) Appearance of interleukin-1 in macrophages and in ramified microglia in the brain of endotoxin-

treated rats: a pathway for the induction of non-specific symptoms of sickness? *Brain Res 588*, 291-6.

[338] Matsumura, K., Kobayashi, S. (2004) Signaling the brain in inflammation: the role of endothelial cells. *Front Biosci 9*, 2819-26.

[339] Langhans, W., Hrupka, B. (1999) Interleukins and tumor necrosis factor as inhibitors of food intake. *Neuropeptides 33*, 415-24.

[340] Soszynski, D. (2004) "Sickness behavior"-mechanisms of origin and significance]. *Postepy Hig Med Dosw 58*, 74-82.

[341] Rittner, H.L., Brack, A., Stein, C. (2002) [Pain and the immune system: friend or foe?]. *Anaesthesist 51*, 351-8.

[342] Schaible, H.G., Richter, F. (2004) Pathophysiology of pain. *Langenbecks Arch Surg 389*, 237-43.

[343] Rao, T.S., Currie, J.L., Shaffer, A.F., Isakson, P.C. (1994) In vivo characterization of zymosan-induced mouse peritoneal inflammation. *J Pharmacol Exp Ther 269*, 917-25.

[344] von Banchet, G.S., Petrow, P.K., Brauer, R., Schaible, H.G. (2000) Monoarticular antigen-induced arthritis leads to pronounced bilateral upregulation of the expression of neurokinin 1 and bradykinin 2 receptors in dorsal root ganglion neurons of rats. *Arthritis Res 2*, 424-7.

[345] Natorska, J., Plytycz, B. (2005) Strain-specific differences on modulatory effects of morphine on peritoneal inflammation in mice. *Folia Biol (Krakow) 53,* 189-195.

[346] Plytycz, B., Natorska, J. (2002) Morphine attenuates pain and prevents inflammation in experimental peritonitis. *Trends Immunol 23*, 345-6.

[347] Cabot, P.J. (2001) Immune-derived opioids and peripheral antinociception. *Clin Exp Pharmacol Physiol 28*, 230-2.

[348] Brack, A., Rittner, H.L., Machelska, H., Beschmann, K., Sitte, N., Schafer, M., Stein, C. (2004) Mobilization of opioid-containing polymorphonuclear cells by hematopoietic growth factors and influence on inflammatory pain. *Anesthesiology 100*, 149-57.

[349] Machelska, H. (2003) Functional evidence of pain control by the immune system. *Adv Exp Med Biol 521*, 88-97.

[350] Stein, C., Schafer, M., Machelska, H. (2003) Attacking pain at its source: new perspectives on opioids. *Nat Med 9*, 1003-8.

[351] Chadzinska M, S.K., Scislowska-Czarnecka A, Bilecki W, Pierzchala-Koziec K, Przewlocki R, Przewlocka B, Plytycz B. (2005) Morphine-induced changes in the activity of proopiomelanocortin and prodynorphin systems in zymosan-induced peritonitis in mice. *Immunol Lett 101*, 185-92.

[352] Chadzinska M., S.-C.A., Pierzchala-Koziec K., Plytycz B. (2005) Met-enkephalin involvement in zymosan-induced peritonitis in Swiss mice. *Mediators Inflamm 2005*, 112-7.

[353] Chadzinska, M., Maj, M., Scislowska-Czarnecka, A., Przewlocka, B., Plytycz, B. (2001) Expression of proenkephalin (PENK) mRNA in inflammatory leukocytes during experimental peritonitis in Swiss mice. *Pol J Pharmacol 53*, 715-8.

[354] Chadzinska, M., Scislowska-Czarnecka, A., Pierzchala-Koziec, K., Plytycz, B. (2003) Inflammation-induced alternations in local and central Met-enkephalin in mice. *Pol J Pharmacol 55*, 467-70.

[355] Makman, M.H. (1994) Morphine receptors in immunocytes and neurons. *Adv Neuroimmunol 4*, 69-82.

[356] Jozefowski, S., Plytycz, B. (1997) Characterization of opiate binding sites on the goldfish (*Carassius auratus* L.) pronephric leukocytes. *Pol J Pharmacol 49*, 229-37.

[357] Eisenstein, T.K., Hilburger, M.E. (1998) Opioid modulation of immune responses: effects on phagocyte and lymphoid cell populations. *J Neuroimmunol 83*, 36-44.

[358] Peterson, P.K., Molitor, T.W., Chao, C.C. (1998) The opioid-cytokine connection. *J Neuroimmunol 83*, 63-9.

[359] Amiche, M., Seon, A.A., Wroblewski, H., Nicolas, P. (2000) Isolation of dermatoxin from frog skin, an antibacterial peptide encoded by a novel member of the dermaseptin genes family. *Eur J Biochem 267*, 4583-92.

[360] Stankiewicz E., W.E., Plytycz B. (2004) Mast cells are responsible for the lack of anti-inflammatory effects of morphine in CBA mice. . *Mediators of Inflammation 13*, 365-368.

[361] Kolaczkowska, E., Seljelid, R., Plytycz, B. (2001) Critical role of mast cells in morphine-mediated impairment of zymosan-induced peritonitis in mice. *Inflamm Res 50*, 415-21.

[362] Chadzinska M., K.E., Scislowska-Czarnecka A., Plytycz B., (2004) Effects of macrophage depletion on peritoneal inflammation in Swiss mice, edible frogs and goldfish. *Folia Biol (Krakow) 52*, 225-231.

[363] Chadzinska M., Scislowska-Czarnecka A., Plytycz B. (2004) Dissociated effects of morphine on mediators of zymosan-induced peritonitis in SWISS mice. In *Molecular Biology in Diagnostics of Infectious Diseases and Biotechnology,* SGGW Press, Warsaw, Poland (M. Niemialtowski ed.), 108-111.

[364] Rogers, T.J., Steele, A.D., Howard, O.M., Oppenheim, J.J. (2000) Bidirectional heterologous desensitization of opioid and chemokine receptors. *Ann N Y Acad Sci 917*, 19-28.

[365] Grimm, M.C., Ben-Baruch, A., Taub, D.D., Howard, O.M., Resau, J.H., Wang, J.M., Ali, H., Richardson, R., Snyderman, R., Oppenheim, J.J. (1998) Opiates transdeactivate chemokine receptors: delta and mu opiate receptor-mediated heterologous desensitization. *J Exp Med 188*, 317-25.

[366] Grimm, M.C., Ben-Baruch, A., Taub, D.D., Howard, O.M., Wang, J.M., Oppenheim, J.J. (1998) Opiate inhibition of chemokine-induced chemotaxis. *Ann N Y Acad Sci 840*, 9-20.

[367] Chadzinska, M., Plytycz, B. (2004) Differential migratory properties of mouse, fish, and frog leukocytes treated with agonists of opioid receptors. *Dev Comp Immunol 28*, 949-58.

[368] Bhat, R.S., Bhaskaran, M., Mongia, A., Hitosugi, N., Singhal, P.C. (2004) Morphine-induced macrophage apoptosis: oxidative stress and strategies for modulation. *J Leukoc Biol 75*, 1131-8.

[369] Singhal, P.C., Kapasi, A.A., Franki, N., Reddy, K. (2000) Morphine-induced macrophage apoptosis: the role of transforming growth factor-beta. *Immunology 100*, 57-62.

[370] Kolaczkowska, E., Plytycz, B. (2003) Interstrain and intrastrain differences in peritonitis induced by various doses of zymosan: studies on Balb/c and C57BL/6J mice. In *Molecular Biology in Diagnostics of Infectious Diseases and Biotechnology,* SGGW Press, Warsaw, Poland (M. Niemialtowski ed.), 108-111.

[371] Scislowska-Czarnecka, A., Chadzinska, M., Pierzchala-Koziec, K., Plytycz, B. (2004) Long-lasting effects of social stress on peritoneal inflammation in some strains of mice. *Folia Biol (Krakow) 52*, 97-104.

[372] Stankiewicz, E., Wypasek, E., Plytycz, B. (2001) Opposite effects of mast cell degranulation by compound 48/80 on peritoneal inflammation in Swiss and CBA mice. *Pol J Pharmacol 53*, 149-55.

[373] Plytycz, B., Seljelid, R. (1997) Rhythms of immunity. *Arch Immunol Ther Exp (Warsz) 45*, 157-62.

[374] Plytycz, B., Chadzinska, M., Mika, J., Labuz, D., Przewlocka, B., Przewlocki, R. (1998) Morphine reverses the inhibitory effects of repeated saline injections on peritoneal inflammation in mice. *Pol J Pharmacol 50*, 271-3.

[375] Natorska, J., Chadzinska, M., Scisłowska-Czarnecka, A., Plytycz, B. (2001) Stress of saline injections or aseptic puncture modifies subsequent peritoneal inflammation. In *Molecular Biology in Diagnostics of Infectious Diseases and Biotechnology,* SGGW Press, Warsaw, Poland (M. Niemialtowski ed.), 142-144.

[376] Kolaczkowska, E., Chadzinska, M., Seljelid, R., Plytycz, B. (2001) Strain differences in some immune parameters can be obscured by circadian variations and laboratory routines: studies of male C57BL/6J, Balb/c and CB6 F1 mice. *Lab Anim 35*, 91-100.

[377] Moynihan, J.A., Karp, J.D., Cohen, N., Cocke, R. (1994) Alterations in interleukin-4 and antibody production following pheromone exposure: role of glucocorticoids. *J Neuroimmunol 54*, 51-8.

[378] Ader, R., Cohen, N., Felten, D. (1995) Psychoneuroimmunology: interactions between the nervous system and the immune system. *Lancet 345*, 99-103.

[379] Plytycz, B., Seljelid, R. (2002) Stress and immunity: minireview. *Folia Biol (Krakow) 50*, 181-9.

[380] Plytycz, B., Seljelid, R. (2003) From inflammation to sickness: historical perspective. *Arch Immunol Ther Exp (Warsz) 51*, 105-9.

[381] Kelley, K.W. (2004) From hormones to immunity: the physiology of immunology. *Brain Behav Immun 18*, 95-113.

[382] Dantzer, R. (2004) Innate immunity at the forefront of psychoneuroimmunology. *Brain Behav Immun 18*, 1-6.

[383] Chomczynski, P., Sacchi, N. (1987) Single-step method of RNA isolation by acid guanidinium thiocyanate-phenol-chloroform extraction. *Anal Biochem 162*, 156-9.

[384] Pierzchala, K., Van Loon, G.R. (1990) Plasma native and peptidase-derivable Met-enkephalin responses to restraint stress in rats. Adaptation to repeated restraint. *J Clin Invest 85*, 861-73.

INDEX

A

B

D

E

F

G

H

I

J

K

L

M

N

O

P

S

T